The Health Promoting Cookbook

Simple, Guilt-Free, Vegetarian Recipes

ed. by Alan Goldhamer, D.C.

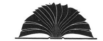

Book Publishing Company
Summertown, Tennessee

© 1997 Alan Goldhamer
Cover design: Bev Lacy
Cover Photos Copyright © 1996 PhotoDisk, Inc.
Interior Design: Cynthia Holzapfel

24 23 22 21   11 12 13

Printed in the United States of America.

Book Publishing Company
P. O. Box 99
Summertown, TN 38483
1-888-260-8458
www.bookpubco.com

ISBN10 1-57067-024-2
ISBN13 978-1-57067-024-4

Library of Congress Cataloging-in-Publication
The health promoting cookbook : simple guilt-free, vegetarian
   recipes/ ed. by Alan Goldhamer.
        p.   cm.
     Includes index.
     ISBN 1-57067-024-2 (alk. paper)
     1. Vegetarian cookery.   I. Goldhamer, Alan.
RM236.H39 1997
641.5'6363--dc21   96-46760
                                                  CIP

BOOK
PUBLISHING
COMPANY

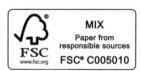

MIX
Paper from
responsible sources
FSC® C005010

We chose to print this title on responsibly harvested paper stock certified by The Forest Stewardship Council, an independent auditor of responsible forestry practices. For more information, visit us.fsc.org.

CONTENTS

Eat to Live

This is a very special and unique cookbook. Most cookbooks are written by and for people who live to eat, but this cookbook is designed for people who want to eat to live—and live healthfully.

The recipes in this book are free of added fat and oil. All recipes completely avoid meat, fish, fowl, eggs, and dairy products, as well as the use of added oil, salt, and sugar. Most of the recipes also avoid the use of glutinous grains such as wheat, rye, and barley. All of the recipes use readily available ingredients derived exclusively from whole natural foods such as fresh fruits and vegetables, whole grains, and legumes.

The Health Promoting Cookbook provides you with a week of "integrated recipes" designed to minimize your time in the kitchen.

Special recipes good for holiday feasts, feeding children, losing weight, and dealing with food sensitivities and allergies are provided.

Detailed nutritional information is included for each recipe as well as a weekly menu, designed to give examples of how you can combine these recipes for optimum nutrition.

Comprehensive shopping lists of all the ingredients and kitchen tools you need to make these recipes are included in the appendix.

This book is designed for individuals who want to make simple, good tasting, health-promoting food. The recipes have been developed and thoroughly taste-tested at the TrueNorth Health Center, a residential health care center in Penngrove, California (see p. 179 for additional information).

The Health
Promoting
Cookbook

Thinking Straight About Food

Eating is one of our most basic and powerful drives. And while eating has been woven into many cultural and religious practices, essentially we eat to survive. There are many basic requirements of life that we can get only through our diet. We need a source of fuel or calories; we need protein, essential fatty acids, vitamins, minerals, fiber, and water.

There are huge industries in this country trying to convince us that it doesn't matter what we eat. We are told that any combination of heated, treated, processed, chemicalized "foods" will meet our nutritional needs so long as we take plenty of vitamin pills, heartburn medicine, and headache remedies.

If these same forces were selling fuel for your car, they would try to convince you that your car would run just fine on any fluid so long as you could get it into the gas tank. Then, when you took your car back to the guy who said that it would run fine on coffee ice cream and you complained of pinging and a fouled up carburetion system, he would keep you waiting for two hours and then tell you that it was "probably all in your head," that you should "learn to live with it," ask "what do you expect at your car's age," then announce "there's nothing that can be done."

Food choices matter

At the turn of the century people died before they reached their genetic potential because of acute diseases. Tuberculosis, pneumonia, and gastrointestinal diseases were leading causes of death. Due to changes in public health measures, improved nutrition, and medical treatment, acute illness is no longer a leading cause of death. Today, people die from chronic degenerative disease.

Atherosclerotic vascular disease is a buildup of fat in the blood vessels, and the associated heart attacks and strokes kill about half of all the people that die each year. Cancer of the breast, colon, prostate, lung, and other organs is associated with 25 percent of all the people that die each year. Diabetes, cirrhosis of the liver, and emphysema also kill many people prematurely.

What do all of these conditions have in common? They are caused or massively influenced by the food choices we make—what we put or don't put into our mouths.

What to avoid and why

Of all the things human beings put in their mouths, tobacco, alcohol, caffeine, recreational and prescription drugs are perhaps the most harmful. The seemingly endless and varied attempts by people to modify their internal chemistry through powerful chemical agents is an ever widening tragedy. In my practice I treat more people who are suffering and dying from the consequences of using and abusing chemicals than I care to think about. We all need to remember that headaches are not caused by an aspirin deficiency and that there are more productive ways of modifying our moods than with pills, potions and elixirs.

Perhaps the second most destructive habit I see is the use of animal products. Meat, fish, fowl, eggs, and dairy products all have much in common. In addition to the well-documented health reasons, there are economic, environmental, humanitarian, and for many, spiritual reasons that support the adoption of a vegetarian diet.

Not designed for meat

Unlike other animals that include meat in their diet, humans are unable to break down uric acid to allantoin. This inability to break down uric acid leads to an increased possibility of it accumulating in the body when animal products are eaten. Uric acid is an intermediary product of metabolism that is associated with various pathological states, including gout.

The human liver, unlike the livers of carnivores, can only process a limited amount of cholesterol. If significant amounts of animal products are consumed, cholesterol levels rise, along with an increased risk of developing atherosclerosis.

Clearly, either we were not designed to eat animal products or we somehow have the wrong kind of liver.

Animal products, such as uncooked or improperly cooked meat, fish, fowl and dairy products, are a source of parasites and contamination. Trichinae, found in pork and pork-contaminated beef, can cause trichinosis. Salmonellae, found in chicken, eggs and other contaminated animal products, can cause salmonellosis. In addition to the above "naturally occurring" problems with animal products, a multitude of chemical agents—such as nitrites, etc.—are added to animal products to slow down their decay, improve their color, and alter their taste.

Chemicals in meat

In addition to parasites, bacterial infestation, toxic poisons, and carcinogenic agents, animal products also pose the problem of biological concentration. Animals consume large quantities of grain, grass, etc., that are, to a greater or lesser extent, contaminated with herbicides, pesticides, and other agents. In addition, animals are often fed antibiotics and treated with other drugs and toxic agents. These poisons concentrate in the fat of the animal and are present in an animal's milk and flesh. This biological concentration of poisons poses significant threats to the health of humans who consume animal products.

As if this weren't enough, animal products are completely devoid of fiber and anti-oxidants and are extremely high in protein—and in spite of what millions of dollars of meat and dairy industry advertising would have you believe, it is excess, not inadequate protein, that is the threat to health. Excess protein has been strongly implicated as a causal agent in many disease processes, including kidney disease, various forms of cancer, increased blood cholesterol, a host of autoimmune and hypersensitivity disease processes, and osteoporosis.

It is ironic that the chief argument used to promote the use of animal products—the purported need for large quantities of protein—is one of the greatest reasons for avoiding them. If animal products are included in the diet in significant quantities, it becomes ever more difficult to ingest adequate quantities of the plant materials known to reduce the risk of chronic degenerative disease.

Fish, fowl, and fat

Because animal products are so high in fat, segments of the "food" industry are advertising their products as "lower" in fat. Because of this advertising, some people want to believe that if they change the color of their meat from red to white or if they remove the skin of the animal before eating it, they can avoid the toxic fat.

If you want to see big changes in your health, you must make big changes in your life. Token changes don't work. Only

dramatic reduction or elimination of all animal products merits your consideration.

Thinking straight about food

A woman was recently referred to me for nutritional counseling by her gynecologist. I reviewed her history, performed a physical examination, and was explaining the dietary recommendations I had prepared for her. She interrupted me and said, "Look, doctor, I knew I was coming here for nutritional advice, but I didn't know I would have to eat differently." Many times patients ask me, "If I have to avoid drugs including alcohol, coffee, cola, and chocolate; animal products including meat, fish, fowl, eggs and dairy products; and oil and refined carbohydrates—what's left?"

The answer is: a diet derived exclusively from whole natural foods—fresh fruits, vegetables, whole grains, and the variable addition of nuts, seeds, and legumes.

Old habits die hard

Why do we find it so difficult to eat what we should eat and avoid what we shouldn't?

Part of it is genetics—we are programmed to eat concentrated foods when they are available. That is an important survival trait. In a natural setting, there are no chocolate chip cookie trees, candy vines, or burger bushes. But today, surrounded by unlimited access to concentrated foods, we must overcome our instincts with our intellect.

To eat well, we have to understand the factors that drive us to eat so poorly. Very often we eat for the wrong reasons. We might eat because we are emotionally distraught. We might feel fatigued and eat for stimulation. But when we are tired, we should sleep.

Fear of being different is another factor that drives us to make poor food choices. "Friends" can experience a lot of cognitive dissonance. "You're no fun anymore!" "It's not healthy to be a fanatic!" "You're so thin!" "Don't you think you're carrying this a little too far!" "I made it just for you!" "A little won't hurt!"

Once at a lecture I gave, a woman in her 80s stood up and told the group that when she was in her 40s she was very ill. Because conventional treatments failed her, as a last resort she tried fasting and changing her diet. It worked! But some of her friends were so critical of her new lifestyle that she eventually stopped seeing them. I asked if she felt that it was a great loss, but she said, "Oh, no dear. They all died years ago."

Your Transition to Healthful Eating

What should you put on your plate when you eat?

The most frequent questions people making a transition to healthful eating ask are: What should I eat to insure that I will meet my body's nutritional needs? What foods and other substances should I avoid? Will I enjoy my new diet and feel good physically and emotionally about it? And can I do it?

The answers to the first two questions have been stated previously—eat a plant-based diet derived exclusively from whole natural foods, and avoid meat, fish, fowl, eggs, and dairy products, as well as added oil, salt, and sugar, and most processed foods. Of course, there is considerable variation in how different individuals approach the *specifics* of diet, but the guiding principles remain the same. The basic challenges we face are these. How do I get enough to eat to meet my individual needs? How do I avoid excess consumption? And how do I avoid the consumption of health compromising foods and other detrimental substances?

Individual needs

People come in all shapes and sizes. We have different metabolisms, different activity levels, different heights and weights, and different ages, each with individual capacities for digestion. And since each of these factors can change during our lifetime, we always need to fashion a diet that meets our individual needs.

With this in mind, I want to give two examples of daily menus, one for a healthy, active 25 to 50-year-old female, the other for a healthy, active 25 to 50-year-old male (shown in the box at right).

Healthful eating strategies

The quantity and quality of needed nutrients, including vitamins and minerals, are clearly provided in abundance by a vegetarian diet. This type of diet also ensures that the percentage of calories derived from fat and protein can be kept within healthful ranges. Another plus is that this type of diet is less stimulating, which dramatically reduces the tendency to overeat.

Since raw fruits and vegetables are such nutrition powerhouses, one might wonder if the entire diet should be derived from raw foods only. In practice, the attempt to live exclusively on raw foods can present some challenges. Raw vegetables contain only about 100 calories per pound, and much of the available energy (calories) in the food is used up in the process of mastication and digestion, as well as eliminating the high fiber content of these foods. If one were to subsist on raw vegetables only, it would clearly be a full-time job. You would literally have to eat all day long (much like most other grazing animals do).

Sample menu for a woman

An example of a health-promoting diet pattern for a healthy, active 25 to 50-year-old female might be:

Breakfast: fresh raw fruit salad including a banana, apple, and strawberries along with celery and one ounce each of almonds and raw pumpkin seeds.

Lunch: large raw vegetable salad (lettuce, carrot, beets, tomato, alfalfa sprouts, peas, and cucumber) with avocado-tomato dressing and a huge plate of steamed vegetables and a baked potato.

Dinner: raw vegetable plate (carrot, jicama, celery, cucumber) with steamed vegetables and brown rice/lentil stew.

Sample menu for a man

An example of a health-promoting diet pattern for a healthy, active 25 to 50-year-old male might be:

Breakfast: orange juice smoothie (orange juice, banana, kiwi) and oatmeal with raisins.

Lunch: vegetable plate with avocado dip, steamed vegetables, and potato/vegetable soup.

Dinner: large raw vegetable salad (lettuce, carrot, beets, tomato, alfalfa sprouts, peas, cucumber) with avocado-tomato dressing a huge plate of steamed vegetables a bowl of split pea/yam soup over brown rice.

If additional calories are required, fresh mixed vegetable juice or fresh fruit could be consumed in the afternoon.

Problems with all-fruit diets

Fruit is more concentrated, providing about 300 calories per pound. Large quantities of fruit could provide adequate calories, but such a diet would be very high in sugar and low in minerals, which would eventually lead to health problems for many, if not most, people. The patients I have seen who have eaten predominantly raw fruit diets for any length of time often develop multiple health problems including difficulties with teeth, gums, skin, immune system, and nervous system. Increased emotional volatility, fatigue, recurrent fungal, yeast, bacterial, and viral infections are also common.

Introducing raw nuts to the raw fruit diet adds a rich source of nutrition. But the resulting high-fat, high-sugar diet does not appear to work as well as a diet that utilizes abundant quantities of fresh fruits and vegetables with the addition of significant quantities of cooked starches such as vegetables, whole grains, and legumes.

Cooked starches are rich sources of nutrients, including minerals. Conservative cooking such as steaming and baking causes minimal degradation of nutrients, and cooked starches contain significantly more available energy per volume than raw foods. The cooking process breaks down the starch and fiber, making the consumption of appropriate quantities of health-promoting food both feasible and practical. The inclusion of high starch foods as a staple of the diet helps insure that we avoid the consumption of unacceptable levels of fat, protein, and/or soluble sugars.

Enjoying your diet

The question of whether or not you will enjoy your new diet is somewhat difficult to answer. When making a swift and dramatic dietary change—from a typical western diet to a health-promoting diet—people sometimes temporarily feel physically worse and emotionally deprived. For a very determined person this method can be an excellent choice, and almost everyone can make at least limited positive changes in this direction.

At the TrueNorth Health Center, we often see people who want or need to make a change rapidly. For these people, a period of therapeutic water fasting followed by a carefully controlled refeeding period speeds the transition. Fasting affects the body in many profound ways. The taste buds are dramatically rejuvenated and the taste of simple food can be truly appreciated. A fast also can enable a person to more quickly get through the sometimes unpleasant physical symptoms associated with detoxification and radical metabolic change. If you would like to receive an information packet about the center, please call (707) 586-5555 or write:

TrueNorth Health Center
6010 Commerce Blvd. #152
Rohnert Park, CA 94928

Living in the real world

We all live in the real world, with its temptations and seductions. Unfortunately, many things that taste good do not promote health. They have been designed to appeal to our inborn (and socially conditioned?) preferences for sweet, salt, and fat. In a natural setting, these substances are scarce, but in our industrial society we have access to virtually unlimited rich, stimulating foods.

To be successful in dietary transition, you must create your own natural environment as much as possible. The most important place to start is your home.

Don't bring fats, oils, salt, and sugar, processed foods or animal products into your home—not even "just for company." If you have these temptations around you, you will either succumb to them or spend so much energy trying to resist them that you will become exhausted.

It is important for each person to develop his or her own set of strategies to support a healthful lifestyle. It is also important to review these strategies as well as your reasons for wanting to live healthfully. Cultivate friends who value their health and happiness. Pursue activities and interests that give you a feeling of productivity and emotional nourishment rather than looking solely to food to make you feel good.

Remember, food is fuel. Eat to live; don't live to eat.

One-Week Menu Plan

The following week of meal plans will provide you with an example of how you can integrate the recipes in this book into a healthful diet plan. The dietary analyses on pp. 18-19 show that these meal plans actually contribute more than 100% of the Recommended Dietary Allowances of various nutrients as established by the National Academy of Science.

Foods for Day 1
Breakfast

	Average 25 to 50 year old female	Average 25 to 50 year old male
orange juice	2 cups	2 cups
cooked oatmeal	3 cups	4 cups
Applesauce, p. 171	1 cup	1 cup

Lunch

raw vegetable salad*	1 serving	1 serving
Tofu Spinach Dip, p. 140	12 ounces	12 ounces

Dinner

raw vegetable salad*	1 serving	1 serving
steamed kale	2 cups	2 cups
Shepherd's Pie, p. 82	1 1/2 servings	2 servings
steamed broccoli	3 cups	3 cups

Foods for Day 2
Breakfast

Home Fries, p. 80	2 servings	2 servings

Lunch

fruit salad**	1 serving	1 serving
Cashew Cream, p. 43	3 1/2 ounces	3 1/2 ounces

Dinner

raw vegetable salad*	1 serving	1 serving
Sweet Scarlet Salad Dressing, p. 67	1 serving	1 serving
Split Pea and Yam Soup, p. 24	1 serving	2 servings
Corn Bread, p. 134	3 servings	3 servings
steamed green beans	3 cups	3 cups

(*, ** see p. 17)

Foods for Day 3
Breakfast

	Average 25 to 50 year old female	Average 25 to 50 year old male
raw fruit salad**	1 serving	1 1/2 servings
raw sunflower seeds	3 ounces	3 ounces

Lunch

raw vegetable salad*	1 serving	1 serving
Potato Salad with Avocado Dressing, p. 138, 68	1 serving	1 serving
Corn Bread (from Day 2)	3 servings	3 servings

Dinner

raw vegetable salad*	1 serving	1 serving
Cucumber Kiwi Dressing, p. 70	1 serving	1 serving
steamed corn on the cob	2 ears	2 ears
Stuffed Peppers, p. 106	2 servings	2 servings

Foods for Day 4
Breakfast

fresh apple juice	2 cups	2 cups
cooked oatmeal	3 cups	4 cups
unsulphured raisins	1/2 cup	1/2 cup

Lunch

Holiday Pear Salad, p. 61	1 serving	1 serving

Dinner

raw vegetable salad*	1 serving	1 serving
Steam-Fry Vegetables, p. 109	1 1/2 servings	1 1/2 servings

(*, ** see p. 17)

Foods for Day 5
Breakfast

	Average 25 to 50 year old female	Average 25 to 50 year old male
cantaloupe	1/2 melon	1/2 melon
honeydew	2 cups	2 cups
watermelon	2 cups	2 cups

Lunch

Oriental Rice Salad, p. 147	1 serving	1 1/2 servings
nori seaweed	1/4 ounce (3 sheets)	1/4 ounce (3 sheets)
Smooth Emerald Soup, p. 39	1 serving	1 1/2 servings

Dinner

raw vegetable salad*	1 serving	1 serving
Avocado Dressing, p. 68	1 serving	1 serving
steamed broccoli	3 cups	3 cups
Polenta Vegetable Casserole, p. 102	1 serving	1 1/2 servings

Foods for Day 6
Breakfast

raw fruit salad**	1 serving	1 1/2 servings
raw pumpkin seeds	3 ounces	3 ounces

Lunch

Chinese Cabbage Salad, p. 55	2 servings	2 servings

Dinner

raw vegetable salad*	1 serving	1 serving
Vegetable Lentil Soup, p. 38	1 serving	1 1/2 servings
cooked long grain brown rice	3 cups	3 cups
corn tortillas	4 tortillas	4 tortillas

(*, ** see p. 17)

Foods for Day 7
Breakfast

	Average 25 to 50 year old female	Average 25 to 50 year old male
Stuffed Baked Apples, p. 170	2 servings	2 servings

Lunch

Yamburgers, p. 113	2 servings	2 servings
No-Fat Fries, p. 142	2 servings	2 servings
Homemade Ketchup, p. 49	1 serving	1 serving

Dinner

raw vegetable salad*	1 serving	1 serving
Sweet Scarlet Salad Dressing, p. 67	1 serving	1 serving
Corn Pasta, p. 96	2 servings	2 1/2 servings
Vegetable Marinara Sauce, p. 47	1 serving	1 serving
steamed spinach	2 cups	2 cups

*One Serving Raw Vegetable Salad

Romaine Lettuce	2 cups
Celery	1 cup
Carrots	1 cup
Tomato	1 small
Peeled Lemon	1/2 lemon

**One Serving Raw Fruit Salad

Banana	1
Orange	1
Strawberries	1
Pear	1

General Dietary Analysis of the One-Week Menu

This chart lists the average daily nutrient content for the week of recipes. The RDA% is the percentage of the recommended daily allowance for an average female 25 to 50 years old. Any specific individual may require more or less total food intake depending on height, weight, age, energy expenditure, etc.

Nutrient	Amount	% RDA	Nutrient	Amount	% RDA
Kilocalories	2113 Kc	96	Vitamin A	7867 RE	983
Protein	68 gm.	135	Beta-Carotene	7073 µg.	n/a
Thiamin B1	3 mg.	269	Riboflavin B2	1.9 mg.	146
Cystine	845 mg.	199	Niacin B3	23 mg.	155
Glutamic Acid	229 mg.	n/a	Pyridoxine B6	4.2 mg.	260
Glycine	48 mg.	n/a	Pant. Acid	9 mg.	166
Histidine	1394 mg.	254	Cobalamine B12	0 µg.	0*
Isoleucine	2494 mg.	384	Folate	934 µg.	519
Leucine	4259 mg.	448	Vitamin C	605 mg.	1008
Lysine	2914 mg.	364	Vitamin E	25 mg.	310
Methionine	950 mg.	223	Vitamin K	1000 µg.	1538
Phenylalanine	2620 mg.	552	Calcium	856 mg.	107
Proline	84 mg.	n/a	Chromium	.22 mg.	176
Serine	51 mg.	n/a	Copper	3.8 mg.	170
Threonine	2133 mg.	474	Iron	28 mg.	187
Tryptophan	707 mg.	283	Magnesium	852 mg.	304
Tyrosine	1804 mg.	380	Manganese	11 mg.	309
Valine	3084 mg.	474	Molybdenum	167 µg.	102
Fat	37 gm.	n/a	Phosphorus	1905 mg.	238
Potassium	7906 mg.	395	Cholesterol	0 mg.	n/a
Selenium	.125 mg.	227	Linoleic Fat	13.9 gm.	284
Sodium	531 mg.	n/a	Linolenic Fat	.3 gm.	n/a
Zinc	12.8 mg	106	Mono Fat	11.5 gm.	n/a
Dietary Fiber	69 gm.	315	Poly Fat	15.7 gm.	n/a
Insoluble Fiber	16 gm.	n/a	Saturated Fat	5.4 gm.	n/a
Soluble Fiber	4.4 gm.	n/a	Carbohydrate	411 gm	149
Weight	3339 gm.	n/a	Sugar	122 gm.	n/a
Caffeine	0 mg.	n/a	Fructose	36 gm.	n/a
Moisture	2790 gm.	n/a	Lactose	0 gm.	n/a
Sucrose	31 gm.	n/a	Glucose	27 gm.	n/a
Alcohol	0 gm.	n/a			

Percent of Calories from: Protein: 12, Fat: 15, Carbohydrates: 73

n/a = not applicable or no standard established   * see p. 20

General Dietary Analysis of the One-Week Menu

This chart lists the average daily nutrient content for the week of recipes. The RDA% is the percentage of the recommended daily allowance for an average male 25 to 50 years old. Any specific individual may require more or less total food intake depending on height, weight, age, energy expenditure, etc.

Nutrient	Amount	% RDA	Nutrient	Amount	% RDA
Kilocalories	2466 Kc	85	Vitamin A	8546 RE	854
Protein	79 gm.	125	Beta-Carotene	7743 µg.	n/a
Thiamin B1	3.4 mg.	226	Riboflavin B2	2.2 mg.	126
Cystine	1012 mg.	189	Niacin B3	26 mg.	139
Glutamic Acid	243 mg.	n/a	Pyridoxine B6	4.8 mg.	239
Glycine	50 mg.	n/a	Pant. Acid	10.5 mg.	191
Histidine	1667 mg.	240	Cobalamine B12	0 µg.	0*
Isoleucine	2915 mg.	356	Folate	1074 µg.	523
Leucine	5081 mg.	424	Vitamin C	673 mg.	1120
Lysine	3446 mg.	342	Vitamin E	28 mg.	284
Methionine	1112 mg.	208	Vitamin K	1066 µg.	1333
Phenylalanine	3113 mg.	520	Calcium	931 mg.	116
Proline	85 mg.	n/a	Chromium	.24 mg.	195
Serine	53 mg.	n/a	Copper	4.4 mg.	197
Threonine	2506 mg.	442	Iron	31 mg.	314
Tryptophan	827 mg.	262	Magnesium	968 mg.	277
Tyrosine	2131 mg.	356	Manganese	12 mg.	354
Valine	3616 mg.	442	Molybdenum	200 µg.	122
Fat	40.51 gm.	n/a	Phosphorus	2174 mg.	272
Potassium	8824 mg.	441	Cholesterol	0 mg.	n/a
Selenium	.145 mg.	207	Linoleic Fat	15.3 gm.	237
Sodium	566 mg.	n/a	Linolenic Fat	.3 gm.	n/a
Zinc	15 mg	100	Mono Fat	12 gm.	n/a
Dietary Fiber	79 gm.	272	Poly Fat	17 gm.	n/a
Insoluble Fiber	18 gm.	n/a	Saturated Fat	5.9 gm.	n/a
Soluble Fiber	5.3 gm.	n/a	Carbohydrate	485 gm	133
Weight	3864 gm.	n/a	Sugar	141 gm.	n/a
Caffeine	0 mg.	n/a	Fructose	42 gm.	n/a
Moisture	3221 gm.	n/a	Lactose	0 gm.	n/a
Sucrose	36 gm.	n/a	Glucose	31 gm.	n/a
Alcohol	0 gm.	n/a			

Percent of Calories from: Protein: 12, Fat: 14, Carbohydrates: 74

n/a = not applicable or no standard established   * see p. 20

Vitamin B12

Vitamin B12 (cobalamin) is produced only by bacteria. A strictly vegan diet (no animal foods) contains only trace amounts of vitamin B12 from bacterial contamination. Some vitamin B12 is produced by the bacteria in our mouth and intestinal tract, but it has not yet been proven that this is adequate for all people. To insure that internal production and recycling of vitamin B12 is adequate, I recommend that vegetarians have a simple blood or urine test every 1-3 years for methylmalonic acid. This is the most sensitive indicator of vitamin B12 status. If the test for methylmalonic acid is positive, inclusion of vitamin B12 fortified foods or oral supplements can be undertaken. Pregnant and lactating mothers should insure themselves of a reliable, vegetarian source of vitamin B12 in their diet, such as Vitamin B12 fortified foods or oral supplementation.

SOUPS

THICK AND SWEET ROSEMARY MILLET SOUP

preparation time: 30 min.
cooking time: 25 min.

servings: 9

12 cups vegetable stock or water
2 cups uncooked millet
2 cups diced celery

1 acorn squash, (2 cups) seeds
removed, sliced in eighths, and
steamed until tender
(about 15 minutes)

2 cups broccoli florets and peeled,
sliced stems
2 cups chopped cauliflower
2 cups diced carrots

4 cups (one bunch) spinach or kale,
chopped
1 Tbsp. rosemary
2 tsp. oregano
2 tsp. garlic powder

❑ Bring stock or water to a boil. Add the millet and celery, and return to a boil for 10 minutes.

❑ Scoop out the flesh from the acorn squash, mash with a fork, and stir into the soup.

❑ Stir in the broccoli, cauliflower, and carrots, and return to a boil for 10 minutes.

❑ Stir in the spinach, rosemary, oregano, and garlic, and continue cooking for 5 minutes.

All information is per serving:

Calories: 254 (14% from protein, 9% from fat)
Protein: 9 gm., Fat: 2.5 gm., Linoleic Acid: 1.0 gm., Fiber: 12.7 gm.
Calcium: 130 mg., Sodium: 87 mg., Iron: 3.2 mg.
B-Carotene: 1403 µg., Vitamin C: 60 mg., Vitamin E: 5.1 mg.
Selenium: .002 mg., Zinc: 1.4 mg.

Mild Winter Soup

preparation time: 20 min.
cooking time: 30 min.

servings: 4

☐ Dice the yams and vegetables into small pieces, and place in an 8-quart soup pot.

☐ Fill the pot with soup stock to two-thirds the depth of the vegetables. Bring to a boil and simmer until all the ingredients are well cooked (approximately 30 minutes), adding more water or stock as needed.

☐ Purée in a food processor. Serve hot.

4 large yams
1/2 head cauliflower
1/2 head broccoli
6 button mushrooms
4 chard leaves

soup stock or water

All information is per serving:

Calories: 150 (15% from protein, 3% from fat)
Protein: 6 gm., Fat: .6 gm., Linoleic Acid: .1 gm., Fiber: 8 gm.
Calcium: 81 mg., Sodium: 97 mg., Iron: 2.0 mg.
B-Carotene: 2555 μg., Vitamin C: 133 mg., Vitamin E: 5.5 mg.
Selenium: .011 mg., Zinc: 1.0 mg.

SPLIT PEA AND YAM SOUP

preparation time: 15 min.
cooking time: 1 hour, 10 min.

servings: 7

9 cups soup stock or water
2 cups dry split peas
3 large yams, peeled and diced
2 potatoes, peeled and diced

3 ribs celery, diced
1 yellow onion, chopped, or 1 Tbsp.
dried flakes
1 Tbsp. garlic powder
1 tsp. dill
1/2 tsp. oregano
1/2 tsp. thyme
2 bay leaves

❑ Bring the soup stock or water and split peas to a boil while preparing the other ingredients. Add the yams and potatoes, and simmer for 30 minutes, stirring occasionally.

❑ Add the celery, onion, and spices, and simmer until the peas are tender (about 30 minutes). Remove the bay leaves.

❑ If a smooth texture is desired, blend in a food processor until smooth.

All information is per serving:
Calories: 294 (21% from protein, 2% from fat)
Protein: 16 gm., Fat: .8 gm., Linoleic Acid: .3 gm., Fiber: 5.1 gm.
Calcium: 71 mg., Sodium: 40.1 mg., Iron: mg. 3.3
B-Carotene: 1068 µg., Vitamin C: 20 mg., Vitamin E: 2.5 mg.
Selenium: .002 mg., Zinc: 2.1 mg.

RED PEPPER PURÉE SOUP

preparation time: 20 min.
cooking time: 50 min.

servings: 6

❑ Combine all the ingredients in an 8-quart soup pot, and bring to a boil. Reduce the heat to medium, and simmer for 45 minutes, or until the potatoes and peppers are tender.

❑ Drain the vegetables, reserving the liquid in a separate bowl. Purée the vegetables in a food processor or blender until very smooth.

❑ Return the purée to the soup pot, and add 1 cup of the reserved liquid back to reach a desired consistency.

❑ Save the remaining liquid as soup stock for other recipes.

❑ Heat the soup on medium-low until just hot (about 5 minutes). Garnish with parsley and thin slices of red pepper, and serve.

12 cups soup stock
6 red potatoes, washed and chopped
8 red bell peppers, cored and chopped
2 cloves garlic, minced, or 1 tsp. garlic powder
fresh parsley, chopped
red pepper strips, for garnish

All information is per serving:

Calories: 145 (9% from protein, 2% from fat)
Protein: 3.3 gm., Fat: 3 gm., Linoleic Acid: .1 gm., Fiber: 2.6 gm.
Calcium: 31 mg., Sodium: 23 mg., Iron: .9 mg.
B-Carotene: 52 µg., Vitamin C: 83 mg., Vitamin E: 7 mg.
Selenium: .001 mg., Zinc: .6 mg.

ROASTED CARROT AND GREEN BEAN PURÉE

preparation time: 35 min.
cooking time: 1 hour, 10 min.

servings: 6

12 cups sliced carrots (1/4 inch thick)
8 cups sliced green beans (1 inch long)
4 cups sliced zucchini (1/4 inch thick)
2 cups water, stock, or celery juice

❑ Place the vegetables and liquid in a 4-quart casserole dish. Cover and roast at 350° F for 45 minutes.

❑ Remove and blend in a food processor with enough additional liquid for a desired consistency.

❑ Reheat in the baking dish for approximately 10 minutes before serving.

Hint: Good over corn pasta or any grain.

All information is per serving:

Calories: 294 (11% from protein, 4% from fat)

Protein: 9.1 gm., Fat: 1.4 gm., Linoleic Acid: .5 gm., Fiber: 17.5 gm.

Calcium: 243 mg., Sodium: 327 mg., Iron: 5.5 mg.

B-Carotene: 11,866 µg., Vitamin C: 33 mg., Vitamin E: 1.5 mg.

Selenium: .005 mg., Zinc: 2.3 mg.

RUTH'S YAM SOUP

preparation time: 15 min.
cooking time: 60 min.

servings: 6

❑ Bring the liquid to a boil in an 8-quart pot. Add all the ingredients, except the fresh corn. Lower the heat to medium, and simmer until the vegetables are soft (about 35 minutes).

❑ Remove from the heat and blend in a food processor until smooth. Return to the pot and then add the corn. Cook on low heat for 20 minutes, and serve.

Optional seasonings:
1/2 tsp. cinnamon and 1/2 tsp. ginger, or 1/2 tsp. sage and 1/2 tsp. marjoram, or 1/2 tsp. dill

5 cups water or soup stock
8 cups peeled, chopped yams
2 large carrots, chopped
2 large celery stalks, chopped

2 ears of corn, cut from the cob

All information is per serving:

Calories: 247 (6% from protein, 1% from fat)
Protein: 4.0 gm., Fat: .3 gm., Linoleic Acid: .1 gm., Fiber: 5.6 gm.
Calcium: 46 mg., Sodium: 50 mg., Iron: 1.3 mg.
B-Carotene: 3652 µg., Vitamin C: 27 mg., Vitamin E: 8.4 mg.
Selenium: .002 mg., Zinc: .6 mg.

CREAMY TOMATO SOUP

preparation time: 45 min.
cooking time: 45 min.

servings: 8

4 cups water or soup stock
5 ribs celery, juiced (1 cup), or 1 cup
    stock
3 russet potatoes, peeled and diced
3 Yukon Gold potatoes, diced
1 sweet potato, peeled and diced
10 tomatoes, puréed
1/2 cup tomato paste

8 mushrooms, cleaned and sliced
1 zucchini, sliced
1 Tbsp. basil
1/2 cup apple juice

❑ In an 8-quart soup pot, bring the water, celery juice or stock, white potatoes, sweet potato, tomato purée, and tomato paste to boil.

❑ Cook until the potatoes are soft (approximately 25 minutes), stirring occasionally.

❑ While the potatoes are cooking, steam-fry the mushrooms, zucchini, and basil in the apple juice until the mushrooms are tender (approximately 10 minutes), stirring occasionally.

❑ Add the steamed mixture to the soup pot. Blend the entire soup mix in batches in a food processor until smooth.

❑ Return to the soup pot, and heat thoroughly before serving.

All information is per serving:

Calories: 216 (10% from protein, 4% from fat)

Protein: 5.7 gm., Fat: .9 gm., Linoleic Acid: .4 gm., Fiber: 7.4 gm.

Calcium: 46 mg., Sodium: 180 mg., Iron: 2.9 mg.

B-Carotene: 536 µg., Vitamin C: 61 mg., Vitamin E: 1.6 mg.

Selenium: .004 mg., Zinc: .9 mg.

Yam Soup

preparation time: 25 min.
cooking time: 40 min.

servings: 8

❑ Place the yams, onion, and 5 cups water in an 8-quart soup pot. Bring to a boil, then simmer until the yams are tender (about 20 minutes).

❑ Separate the liquid from the yams, and blend the yams and onions in a food processor until smooth; set aside.

❑ In the reserved liquid, steam-fry the peas or green beans, bell pepper, cauliflower, and ginger until just tender (about 5 minutes).

❑ Add the yam mixture, stir thoroughly, and simmer 10 more minutes to blend flavors. Remove the ginger slices before serving. Serve hot as is or over cooked grains or potatoes.

8 medium yams, peeled and diced
1 large onion, diced
5 cups water plus 2 additional cups water to dilute at the end

2 cups fresh or frozen peas or green beans, unsalted
1 red or green bell pepper, diced
1/2 head cauliflower, broken into small chunks (4 cups)
7 slices fresh gingerroot, or 1/4 tsp. powdered ginger

All information is per serving:

Calories: 157 (11% from protein, 3% from fat)

Protein: 4.7 gm., Fat: .5 gm., Linoleic Acid: .1 gm., Fiber: 4.9 gm.

Calcium: 67 mg., Sodium: 29 mg., Iron: 1.6 mg.

B-Carotene: 2498 µg., Vitamin C: 84 mg., Vitamin E: 5.7 mg.

Selenium: .001 mg., Zinc: .7 mg.

HARVEST MEDLEY SOUP

preparation time: 25 min.
cooking time: 30 min.

servings: 11

8 cups water or vegetable stock
1 medium butternut squash, peeled, seeded, and diced

3 carrots, thinly sliced
3 ribs celery, diced
12 large button mushrooms, sliced
1 bunch broccoli, cut into small florets with stems peeled and diced

1 zucchini, cut lengthwise and sliced
1 yellow crookneck squash, sliced and quartered

1 cup frozen green peas
1 1/2 tsp. garlic granules
1 Tbsp. fresh rosemary leaves
1 1/2 tsp. fresh oregano

❑ Bring the water or vegetable stock and squash to a boil, and continue to simmer for 10 minutes.

❑ Add the carrots, celery, mushrooms, and broccoli, and return to simmer for 10 more minutes.

❑ Add the zucchini and crookneck squash, and return to a simmer for 5 minutes.

❑ Add the peas, garlic, and herbs, and continue to simmer for 5 minutes. Serve immediately.

All information is per serving:

Calories: 99 (15% from protein, 5% from fat)

Protein: 4.3 gm., Fat: .6 gm., Linoleic Acid: .1 gm., Fiber: 6.1 gm.

Calcium: 122 mg., Sodium: 51 mg., Iron: 2.4 mg.

B-Carotene: 634 µg., Vitamin C: 73 mg., Vitamin E: .7 mg.

Selenium: .005 mg., Zinc: .8 mg.

White Bean Soup

preparation time: 30 min.
cooking time: 2 hours, 40 min.

servings: 10

❑ Soak the beans overnight in enough water to cover. Rinse and drain thoroughly.

❑ Add enough water to cover, bring the beans to a boil for 5 minutes, and drain again.

❑ Place the beans and 10 cups of stock or water in an 8-quart soup pot. Simmer while preparing the celery, carrots, and leek.

❑ Add the vegetables, sage, and garlic to the soup, and simmer slowly for 2 hours, or until the beans are tender.

❑ Stir in the tomato paste and apple juice, then simmer for another 30 minutes. Serve.

3 cups dried white beans (Great Northern)

10 cups soup stock or water

4 cups chopped celery
4 cups sliced carrots
1 medium leek, sliced

1 tsp. sage
1 Tbsp. garlic powder

12 oz. tomato paste
1/2 cup apple juice

All information is per serving:

Calories: 292 (22% from protein, 3% from fat)
Protein: 16.6 gm., Fat: 1.2 gm., Linoleic Acid: .4 gm., Fiber: 12.9 gm.
Calcium: 213 mg., Sodium: 190 mg., Iron: 7.3 mg.
B-Carotene: 2354 µg., Vitamin C: 25 mg., Vitamin E: 1.2 mg.
Selenium: .001 mg., Zinc: 2.7 mg.

ACORN SQUASH SOUP

preparation time: 30 min.
cooking time: 45 min.

servings: 8

7 cups stock or water
3 acorn squash, peeled and chopped
2 large carrots, peeled and chopped
1 large yam, peeled and chopped
1 tsp. ground ginger
1 tsp. sage

2 cups fresh or frozen corn kernels

❑ In an 8-quart soup pot, bring the stock or water to a boil, and stir in all the ingredients except the corn. Cook on medium-high heat for 20 minutes, or until the squash is soft.

❑ Blend the soup in batches in a food processor or blender until smooth. Return to the pot, add the corn, and reheat on low for 10 minutes.

All information is per serving:

Calories: 172 (8% from protein, 2% from fat)
Protein: 4.0 gm., Fat: .4 gm., Linoleic Acid: .1 gm., Fiber: 6.0 gm.
Calcium: 104 mg., Sodium: 25 mg., Iron: 2.2 mg.
B-Carotene: 817 µg., Vitamin C: 28 mg., Vitamin E: 1.0 mg.
Selenium: .003 mg., Zinc: .6 mg.

CORN CHOWDER

preparation time: 20 min.
cooking time: 45 min.

servings: 6

❑ In an 8-quart soup pot, place all the ingredients and enough water to cover two-thirds of the vegetables. Bring to a boil, cover, and simmer over medium-high heat for 30 minutes.

❑ Remove from the heat and blend two-thirds of the vegetables in batches in a blender or food processor until smooth. Return to the pot and stir in with the unblended vegetables to mix well.

❑ Serve warm as a soup or over a grain or pasta.

4 russet or Yukon Gold potatoes, peeled and diced
1 yam, peeled and diced
10 mushrooms, cleaned and sliced
4 ribs celery, diced
4 ears fresh corn, kernels removed
1/2 bunch broccoli, cut into small florets with stems peeled and diced

All information is per serving:

Calories: 167 (11% from protein, 5% from fat)
Protein: 4.9 gm., Fat: 1.0 gm., Linoleic Acid: .4 gm., Fiber: 5.1 gm.
Calcium: 31 mg., Sodium: 44 mg., Iron: 1.3 mg.
B-Carotene: 418 µg., Vitamin C: 39 mg., Vitamin E: 1.0 mg.
Selenium: .003 mg., Zinc: .9 mg.

33

EXCELLENT BEAN SOUP

preparation time: 20 min.
cooking time: 3 hours

servings: 12

5 cups water or stock
2 cups dried white or pinto beans

1 Tbsp. basil flakes
1 Tbsp. parsley flakes
4 cups chopped mushrooms
4 cups chopped tomatoes
3 ribs celery, diced
1 bunch spinach, well washed and
   chopped

❑ In an 8-quart soup pot, bring the water or stock and beans to a boil, and simmer over medium heat for 2 hours. Add more water or stock if necessary to keep the beans soupy.

❑ Add the remaining ingredients and continue to cook 1 more hour, or until the beans are tender, stirring occasionally.

All information is per serving:

Calories: 126 (22% from protein, 5% from fat)
Protein: 7.3 gm., Fat: .8 gm., Linoleic Acid: .2 gm., Fiber: 7.1 gm.
Calcium: 67 mg., Sodium: 33 mg., Iron: 3.0 mg.
B-Carotene: 103 µg., Vitamin C: 22 mg., Vitamin E: .4 mg.
Selenium: .006 mg., Zinc: 1.1 mg.

TOMATO LENTIL STEW

preparation time: 15 min.
cooking time: 60 min.

servings: 12

❑ Bring the stock or water to a boil. Add the lentils, return to a boil, then simmer for 30 minutes.

❑ Add the carrots, celery, mushrooms, and tomatoes, and simmer for 15 minutes.

❑ Stir in the corn, tomato paste, and seasonings, and continue simmering for 15 minutes, or until the vegetables are tender.

Variation: Leave out the tomatoes and tomato paste for a tasty, mild soup.

12 cups stock or water
4 cups dried lentils

8 cups chopped carrots
8 ribs celery, chopped
4 cups sliced mushrooms
4 tomatoes, diced

2 ears fresh corn kernels cut from the cob
12 oz. tomato paste
2 tsp. basil
2 tsp. garlic powder
2 tsp. sage

All information is per serving:

Calories: 317 (22% from protein, 4% from fat)
Protein: 18.4 gm., Fat: 1.7 gm., Linoleic Acid: .7 gm., Fiber: 15.8 gm.
Calcium: 135 mg., Sodium: 214 mg., Iron: 7.9 mg.
B-Carotene: 3960 µg., Vitamin C: 34 mg., Vitamin E: .8 mg.
Selenium: .019 mg., Zinc: 3.1 mg.

RUTABAGA POTATO SOUP

preparation time: 20 min.
cooking time: 40 min.

servings: 10

3 russet potatoes, peeled
1 large Yukon Gold potato
1 large yam, peeled
3 carrots, peeled
3 ribs celery
1/4 head cabbage
2 large rutabagas, peeled
10 button mushrooms, washed
water or soup stock as needed

❑ Slice all of the ingredients in a food processor or by hand, and place in an 8-quart soup pot.

❑ Cover the vegetables with the water or stock. Bring to a boil, then simmer for 40 minutes, or until all the vegetables are tender.

❑ For added flavor, add 3-4 cups chopped leftover steamed vegetables. Simmer until hot.

❑ Blend in batches in a food processor until smooth, and serve.

All information is per serving:

Calories: 89 (9% from protein, 2% from fat)
Protein: 2.2 gm., Fat: .2 gm., Linoleic Acid: .1 gm., Fiber: 2.9 gm.
Calcium: 26 mg., Sodium: 69 mg., Iron: .8 mg.
B-Carotene: 827 µg., Vitamin C: 20 mg., Vitamin E: 5.4 mg.
Selenium: .006 mg., Zinc: .4 mg.

Homestyle Stew

preparation time: 15 min.
cooking time: 60 min.

servings: 10

❑ In an 8-quart soup pot, whisk the tomato paste and mashed beans into the stock until smooth.

❑ Add the seasonings and half of the potatoes, and simmer for 30 minutes over medium heat.

❑ With a slotted spoon, remove the potatoes and purée in a blender or food processor with 1 cup of the liquid. Return the potatoes to the soup pot, and stir into the stock to thicken.

❑ Add the remaining potatoes and other vegetables, and simmer over medium-low heat for 30 minutes, or until the vegetables are tender.

1/2 cup tomato paste
1/2 cup cooked mashed beans
6 cups vegetable stock

1 tsp. thyme
1/4 tsp. marjoram
6 unpeeled potatoes, scrubbed and cut in 1-inch chunks

1 cup diced carrots
1 cup sliced celery
1 cup fresh corn kernels
1 clove garlic, minced, or 1 onion, diced (optional)

All information is per serving:

Calories: 284 (10% from protein, 7% from fat)
Protein: 8.0 gm., Fat: 2.4 gm., Linoleic Acid: .3 gm., Fiber: 5.7 gm.
Calcium: 566 mg., Sodium: 66 mg., Iron: 38 mg.
B-Carotene: 599 µg., Vitamin C: 28 mg., Vitamin E: .3 mg.
Selenium: .001 mg., Zinc: 2.6 mg.

EGETABLE LENTIL SOUP

preparation time: 15 min.
cooking time: 60 min.

servings: 5

7 cups water
2 cups dried lentils
1 Tbsp. basil
1 Tbsp. parsley flakes

2 tomatoes, diced
2 cups sliced mushrooms
1/2 bunch spinach, well washed and finely chopped

❑ In a 4-quart saucepan, bring the water to a boil. Lower the heat to medium. Add the lentils, basil, and parsley, and simmer for 30 minutes.

❑ Add the tomatoes, mushrooms, and spinach, and simmer for 30 more minutes.

❑ Blend 1/3 of the soup in a food processor or blender until smooth, and return to the pot. Stir and serve.

All information is per serving:
Calories: 227 (30% from protein, 4% from fat)
Protein: 18 gm., Fat: 1.1 gm., Linoleic Acid: .3 gm., Fiber: 10 gm.
Calcium: 158 mg., Sodium: 64 mg., Iron: 7.3 mg.
B-Carotene: 678 µg., Vitamin C: 59 mg., Vitamin E: 1.2 mg.
Selenium: .020 mg., Zinc: 2.8 mg.

SMOOTH EMERALD SOUP

preparation time: 20 min.
cooking time: 30 min.

servings: 6

❑ In the bottom of a 4-quart saucepan, steam-fry the celery and onions in the apple-celery juice until slightly tender, adding water as needed.

❑ Add the mushrooms and steam-fry for 2 minutes.

❑ Add the yams and enough water to almost reach the top of the vegetables. Simmer for 5 minutes.

❑ Add the broccoli and simmer for another 5 minutes.

❑ Add the spinach and continue to simmer until the vegetables are soft.

❑ Blend the soup in batches in a food processor or blender with enough water to create the consistency you desire.

❑ Return the blended soup to the pot, and heat until serving temperature.

Hint: Excellent over rice.

4 ribs celery (include leaves), diced
2 green onions, sliced
1/4 yellow onion, diced
1 cup apple-celery juice, or plain apple juice

2 cups sliced mushrooms

2 large yams, peeled and diced small

1/2 cup finely chopped broccoli

2 cups bunch spinach, washed well, stems removed, and finely chopped
3 cups water

All information is per serving:

Calories: 81 (11% from protein, 4% from fat)
Protein: 2.4 gm., Fat: .4 gm., Linoleic Acid: .1 gm., Fiber: 3.0 gm.
Calcium: 55 mg., Sodium: 51 mg., Iron: 1.4 mg.
B-Carotene: 986 µg., Vitamin C: 45 mg., Vitamin E: 2.3 mg.
Selenium: .004 mg., Zinc: .5 mg.

SAUCES

BARBECUE SAUCE

preparation time: 10 min.
cooking time: 60 min.

servings: 12

12 oz. tomato paste
2 cups apple juice
1/2 cup apple cider vinegar
2 Tbsp. dry mustard
1 Tbsp. minced shallots, or 1 Tbsp.
  garlic powder
1 Tbsp. cinnamon
3 whole star anise (optional)

❑ Combine all the ingredients in a heavy-bottomed saucepan. Cover and cook for one hour over medium-low heat, stirring occasionally. Remove the anise before serving.

Hints: Double or triple this recipe as it will keep covered in the refrigerator for 2-3 weeks. Whole star anise can be found in the spice aisle of your grocery store.

All information is per serving:

Calories: 60 (11% from protein, 12% from fat)
Protein: 1.9 gm., Fat: .9 gm., Linoleic Acid: .2 gm., Fiber: 1.6 gm.
Calcium: 33 mg., Sodium: 23 mg., Iron: 1.7 mg.
B-Carotene: .4 µg., Vitamin C: 14 mg., Vitamin E: n/a
Selenium: .001 mg., Zinc: .4 mg.

CASHEW CREAM

soaking time: 30 min.
preparation time: 15 min.

servings: 6

❑ Soak the ground cashews in the water for 30 minutes. Liquefy the soaked cashews, dates, and vanilla in a blender or food processor.

❑ Add the mango pieces, and blend one at a time, to thicken. Use as a rich sauce.

6 oz. raw cashews, ground (3/4 cup)
1 cup water
4 dates, pitted and minced
1/4 tsp. pure vanilla extract (alcohol-free)

1/4 cup frozen mango pieces

All information is per serving:

Calories: 202 (12% from protein, 58% from fat)
Protein: 6.3 gm., Fat: 13 gm., Linoleic Acid: .01 gm., Fiber: 3.0 gm.
Calcium: 18 mg., Sodium: 7.6 mg., Iron: 2.3 mg.
B-Carotene: 134 µg., Vitamin C: 27 mg., Vitamin E: .8 mg.
Selenium: n/a, Zinc: 1.4 mg.

SWEET AND SOUR SAUCE

preparation time: 15 min.
cooking time: 30 min.

servings: 6

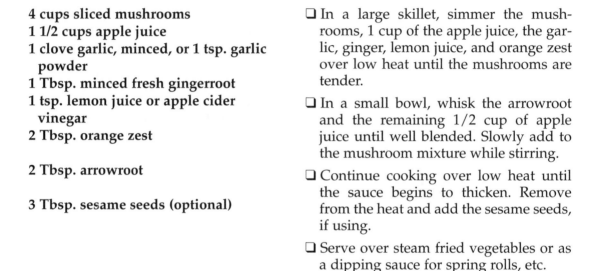

4 cups sliced mushrooms
1 1/2 cups apple juice
1 clove garlic, minced, or 1 tsp. garlic powder
1 Tbsp. minced fresh gingerroot
1 tsp. lemon juice or apple cider vinegar
2 Tbsp. orange zest

2 Tbsp. arrowroot

3 Tbsp. sesame seeds (optional)

❑ In a large skillet, simmer the mushrooms, 1 cup of the apple juice, the garlic, ginger, lemon juice, and orange zest over low heat until the mushrooms are tender.

❑ In a small bowl, whisk the arrowroot and the remaining 1/2 cup of apple juice until well blended. Slowly add to the mushroom mixture while stirring.

❑ Continue cooking over low heat until the sauce begins to thicken. Remove from the heat and add the sesame seeds, if using.

❑ Serve over steam fried vegetables or as a dipping sauce for spring rolls, etc.

All information is per serving:

Calories: 79 (9% from protein, 27% from fat)
Protein: 1.9 gm., Fat: 2.5 gm., Linoleic Acid: 1.0 gm., Fiber: 1.6 gm.
Calcium: 56 mg., Sodium: 4.3 mg., Iron: 1.5 mg.
B-Carotene: .9 µg., Vitamin C: 5.5 mg., Vitamin E: .2 mg.
Selenium: .007 mg., Zinc: .7 mg.

RICH RED SAUCE

preparation time: 15 min.
cooking time: 30 min.

servings: 6

❑ In a 4-quart saucepan, steam-fry the mushrooms, apple juice, and spices for 10 minutes.

❑ Add the tomatoes and simmer 15 more minutes.

❑ Mix the arrowroot with the rice or soy milk, and add slowly to sauce while stirring. Allow the sauce to slowly boil until thick (3-5 minutes).

❑ Serve over pasta or spaghetti squash.

4 cups cleaned, sliced mushrooms
1 cup apple juice
1 Tbsp. Italian seasoning
1/2 tsp. oregano
1/2 tsp. basil
1 Tbsp. garlic powder (optional)

4 cups diced tomatoes

2 Tbsp. arrowroot
1 cup Rice Milk (see p. 151) or low-fat soymilk

All information is per serving:

Calories: 96 (12% from protein, 7% from fat)
Protein: 3.2 gm., Fat: .8 gm., Linoleic Acid: .3 gm., Fiber: 2.4 gm.
Calcium: 57 mg., Sodium: 264 mg., Iron: 2.0 mg.
B-Carotene: 181 μg., Vitamin C: 26 mg., Vitamin E: .5 mg.
Selenium: .014 mg., Zinc: .8 mg.

ZESTY TOMATO SAUCE

preparation time: 15 min.
cooking time: 30 min.

servings: 12

24 oz. tomato paste
6 cups water
1/4 cup apple juice
1 red or green bell pepper, diced or
   sliced in strips
10 mushrooms, cleaned and sliced
3 tomatoes, diced
2 tsp. Italian seasoning
2 tsp. basil
2 tsp. oregano
1 Tbsp. garlic powder
4 bay leaves

❑ Simmer all the ingredients in a medium saucepan at least 30 minutes, stirring occasionally.

All information is per serving:

Calories: 66 (15% from protein, 9% from fat)
Protein: 2.9 gm., Fat: .7 gm., Linoleic Acid: .3 gm., Fiber: 3.2 gm.
Calcium: 41 mg., Sodium: 44 mg., Iron: 2.4 mg.
B-Carotene: 38 µg., Vitamin C: 36 mg., Vitamin E: .2 mg.
Selenium: .002 mg., Zinc: .7 mg.

VEGETABLE MARINARA SAUCE

preparation time: 20 min.
cooking time: 60 min.

servings: 12

❑ In an 8-quart soup pot, bring 3 cups soup stock or water to a boil. Add the eggplant, mushrooms, zucchini, leeks, and bell pepper. Simmer on low heat until tender.

❑ Stir in the tomato paste and remaining stock/water, then add the seasonings. Simmer on low at least an hour, longer if possible.

❑ Add the apple juice and tomatoes for the last 30 minutes of cooking time. The sauce will be chunky; it can be blended in a food processor or blender after cooking if a smooth consistency is desired.

Hint: Good over pasta, rice, or any grain.

6 cups soup stock or water
1 eggplant, cubed
4 cups sliced mushrooms
3 medium zucchini, sliced
2 leek bulbs, chopped
1 red or green bell pepper, chopped

16 oz. tomato paste
3 Tbsp. basil
1 Tbsp. oregano
1 Tbsp. garlic powder
1/2 tsp. rosemary

1 cup apple juice
4 ripe tomatoes, chopped

All information is per serving:

Calories: 85 (13% from protein, 7% from fat)
Protein: 3.2 gm., Fat: .8 gm., Linoleic Acid: .3 gm., Fiber: 3.9 gm.
Calcium: 45 mg., Sodium: 43 mg., Iron: 2.6 mg.
B-Carotene: 57 µg., Vitamin C: 36 mg., Vitamin E: .4 mg.
Selenium: .004 mg., Zinc: .7 mg.

MUSHROOM PEPPER SAUCE

preparation time: 20 min.
cooking time: 30 min.

servings: 4

4 cups sliced mushrooms
2 cups chopped red or green bell
   peppers
1 cup soup stock or celery juice
1/2 cup apple juice

1 tsp. sage
1/2 cup green onions, chopped
2 cups Rice Milk (see p. 151) or low-fat
   soymilk
1 Tbsp. arrowroot

❑ Steam-fry the mushrooms and peppers in the stock and apple juice until tender.

❑ Stir in the sage and green onions, then let simmer while combining rice or soymilk and arrowroot.

❑ Slowly pour the arrowroot mixture into the vegetables, stirring constantly and adding only enough to make a saucy consistency. Save any remaining liquid for thinning the sauce when reheating.

Hint: This sauce has its best flavor when made in advance and allowed to set so the flavors will meld.

All information is per serving:

Calories: 113 (9% from protein, 6% from fat)
Protein: 2.8 gm., Fat: .8 gm., Linoleic Acid: .3 gm., Fiber: 3.3 gm.
Calcium: 25 mg., Sodium: 9 mg., Iron: 1.2 mg.
B-Carotene: 95 µg., Vitamin C: 103 mg., Vitamin E: 1.2 mg.
Selenium: .022 mg., Zinc: .6 mg.

HOMEMADE KETCHUP

preparation time: 10 min.

servings: 12

❑ Combine all the ingredients well in a blender, and store in a covered jar in the refrigerator.

1 cup water
12 oz. tomato paste
2 Tbsp. apple juice
1 Tbsp. lemon juice
1/8 tsp. oregano
1 tsp. onion powder (optional)
1 Tbsp. apple cider vinegar (optional)

All information is per serving:

Calories: 30 (14% from protein, 8% from fat)
Protein: 1.3 gm., Fat: .3 gm., Linoleic Acid: .1 gm., Fiber: 1.4 gm.
Calcium: 13 mg., Sodium: 22 mg., Iron: 1 mg.
B-Carotene: n/a, Vitamin C: 15 mg., Vitamin E: n/a
Selenium: n/a, Zinc: .3 mg.

ENCHILADA SAUCE

preparation time: 10 min.
cooking time: 30 min.

servings: 8

4 1/2 cups water or stock
18 oz. tomato paste
1 cup minced celery
1 1/2 tsp. cumin
1 tsp. coriander or cilantro
1 tsp. garlic powder
1/2 tsp. dry mustard

❑ Whisk the water and tomato paste in a 2-quart saucepan over medium-high heat. Add the remaining ingredients, stirring to mix well.

❑ Lower the heat to medium-low, cover, and simmer for 30 minutes, stirring occasionally.

All information is per serving:

Calories: 69 (16% from protein, 10% from fat)

Protein: 3.2 gm., Fat: .9 gm., Linoleic Acid: .3 gm., Fiber: 3.4 gm.

Calcium: 41 mg., Sodium: 66 mg., Iron: 2.6 mg.

B-Carotene: 3 µg., Vitamin C: 33 mg., Vitamin E: .1 mg.

Selenium: .001 mg., Zinc: .7 mg.

EMERALD SAUCE

preparation time: 15 min.
cooking time: 30 min.

servings: 6

❑ Simmer all the ingredients in a 4-quart saucepan until the carrots and celery are tender (about 15 minutes). Purée in a food processor or blender until smooth, and return to the saucepan. Simmer on low an additional 15 minutes.

Hint: Use on steamed vegetables or mashed potatoes.

2 carrots, peeled and chopped
2 ribs celery, chopped
1 bunch spinach or chard, well washed and stems removed
2 medium tomatoes, chopped
1 Tbsp. basil
1 tsp. garlic powder (optional)
1 cup stock or water

All information is per serving:
Calories: 34 (19% from protein, 6% from fat)
Protein: 1.9 gm., Fat: .3 gm., Linoleic Acid: .1 gm., Fiber: 2.6 gm.
Calcium: 50 mg., Sodium: 129 mg., Iron: 1.7 mg.
B-Carotene: 905 µg., Vitamin C: 22 mg., Vitamin E: 1.2 mg.
Selenium: .024 mg., Zinc: .3 mg.

SALADS AND DRESSINGS

JICAMA-MILLET DINNER SALAD

preparation time: 30 min.
cooking time: 30 min.

servings: 8

1 1/2 cups carrot-celery juice or other liquid
2/3 cup uncooked millet

1 bunch broccoli

1 head romaine lettuce, torn into small pieces
1 small handful fresh cilantro, chopped
1 small handful fresh basil, chopped
4 cups peeled, finely diced jicama, or 4 cups diced water chestnuts
1 carrot, peeled and finely diced
1 cucumber, peeled, sliced, and quartered
1 large handful clover or alfalfa sprouts
1 avocado, diced

❑ Bring the liquid to a boil. Add the millet and return to a boil, then simmer for 30 minutes. Transfer to a mixing bowl, and let cool to room temperature.

❑ Steam the broccoli, then set aside and let cool to room temperature.

❑ Toss together the lettuce, cilantro, basil, jicama, carrot, cucumber, clover sprouts, and avocado.

❑ Cut the broccoli into florets; peel and finely chop the stems. Add the broccoli and millet to the salad, and toss well. Serve cool, but not cold.

All information is per serving:

Calories: 143 (12% from protein, 29% from fat)

Protein: 4.7 gm., Fat: 4.8 gm., Linoleic Acid: .8 gm., Fiber: 6.3 gm.

Calcium: 50 mg., Sodium: 36 mg., Iron: 1.7 mg.

B-Carotene: 1703 µg., Vitamin C: 42 mg., Vitamin E: .7 mg.

Selenium: .001 mg., Zinc: .8 mg.

CHINESE CABBAGE SALAD

preparation time: 20 min.

servings: 6

❑ Wash and dry the cabbage; cut up eight of the leaves, and place in a large mixing bowl. Place the remaining eight leaves on six dinner plates.

❑ Place the avocado, peppers, tomatoes, and grapefruit juice with the cabbage in the mixing bowl. Gently toss and spoon onto the cabbage leaves on the dinner plates.

16 leaves Chinese cabbage (1 cabbage)

2 avocados, quartered, peeled, and diced

2 red or green bell peppers, diced
1 pint cherry tomatoes, cut in half, or 3 medium tomatoes, diced
juice of 1 grapefruit

All information is per serving:

Calories: 172 (11% from protein, 49% from fat)
Protein: 5.2 gm., Fat: 10.7 gm., Linoleic Acid: 1.2 gm., Fiber: 8.2 gm.
Calcium: 104 mg., Sodium: 48 mg., Iron: 1.7 mg.
B-Carotene: 83 µg., Vitamin C: 148 mg., Vitamin E: 1.7 mg.
Selenium: .001 mg., Zinc: .6 mg.

QUINOA AND BLACK BEAN SALAD

preparation time: 30 min.
cooking time: 20 min.
chilling time: 2 hours

servings: 4

1/2 cup soup stock or water
1/4 cup quinoa, well rinsed

1/2 tsp. cumin

2 Tbsp. lemon juice
1/4 cup soup stock
2 Tbsp. minced cilantro
1/2 cup cooked black beans
1 cup fresh corn kernels (2 ears)
1 medium tomato, diced
2 Tbsp. chopped red onion

❑ In a 2-quart saucepan, bring the liquid, quinoa, and cumin to a boil. Cover and reduce the heat to low; cook for 20 minutes or until tender. Remove from the heat and uncover.

❑ In a medium bowl, combine the lemon juice, stock, cilantro, beans, corn, tomato, onion, and cooked quinoa, and stir well.

❑ Chill at least 2 hours, and serve as is or over a bed of lettuce.

All information is per serving:

Calories: 123 (15% from protein, 10% from fat)
Protein: 5.0 gm., Fat: 1.4 gm., Linoleic Acid: .5 gm., Fiber: 3.4 gm.
Calcium: 21 mg., Sodium: 14 mg., Iron: 2.0 mg.
B-Carotene: 35 µg., Vitamin C: 12 mg., Vitamin E: .1 mg.
Selenium: .001 mg., Zinc: .8 mg.

CARROT-RAISIN-RICE SALAD

preparation time: 15 min.
cooking time: 60 min.

servings: 6

❑ In a 2-quart saucepan, bring the water to a boil, add the various types of rice, and return to a boil. Lower the heat and simmer for 45 minutes.

❑ Remove from the heat, add the carrots and spinach, then replace the lid. Allow to stand for 15 minutes. Transfer to a mixing bowl, add the raisins, and fluff with a fork.

3 cups water
3/4 cup short grain brown rice
3/4 cup brown basmati rice
1/2 cup wild rice

2 carrots, grated
1/2 bunch spinach, well washed and chopped
1/2 cup raisins

All information is per serving:

Calories: 273 (10% from protein, 5% from fat)
Protein: 7.1 gm., Fat: 1.6 gm., Linoleic Acid: .5 gm., Fiber: 3.7 gm.
Calcium: 72 mg., Sodium: 38 mg., Iron: 2.5 mg.
B-Carotene: 877 µg., Vitamin C: 6 mg., Vitamin E: 1.1 mg.
Selenium: .012 mg., Zinc: 2.1 mg.

SWEET CARROT SALAD

preparation time: 15 min.
cooking time: 5 min.
chilling time: 1 hour

servings: 3

6 carrots, thinly sliced

2 apples, peeled and diced
1 Tbsp. apple juice
juice of 1 lemon
1/2 tsp. cinnamon
1/2 cup raisins

❑ Steam the carrots for 5 minutes.

❑ Mix all the ingredients in a medium bowl. Chill the salad for 1 hour before serving.

All information is per serving:

Calories: 188 (5% from protein, 3% from fat)
Protein: 2.4 gm., Fat: .7 gm., Linoleic Acid: .2 gm., Fiber: 5.9 gm.
Calcium: 59 mg., Sodium: 53 mg., Iron: 1.5 mg.
B-Carotene: 4054 μg., Vitamin C: 20 mg., Vitamin E: 1.0 mg.
Selenium: .005 mg., Zinc: .4 mg.

MIDEAST GARBANZO BEAN SALAD

preparation time: 20 min.
cooking time: 2 hours
chilling time: 1 hour

servings: 8

❑ Soak the beans overnight in enough water to cover. Rinse well, place in a large saucepan, and add enough water to cover the beans. Bring the beans to a boil, then drain.

❑ Add the 8 cups of water, juice from 1 lemon, and half of the spices, and simmer for 2 hours, or until the beans are tender.

❑ Drain the water, then let the beans cool to room temperature. Add the vegetables, remaining spices, and lemon juice.

❑ Combine well and chill.

3 cups dried garbanzo beans

8 cups water
juice of 3 lemons
2 Tbsp. parsley flakes
1 Tbsp. basil
garlic powder to taste

3 tomatoes, diced
3 ribs celery, diced
1 cucumber, peeled and diced

All information is per serving:

Calories: 297 (21% from protein, 11% from fat)
Protein: 16.6 gm., Fat: 3.9 gm., Linoleic Acid: .1 gm., Fiber: 1.1 gm.
Calcium: 151 mg., Sodium: 46 mg., Iron: 6.1 mg.
B-Carotene: 55 µg., Vitamin C: 24 mg., Vitamin E: .3 mg.
Selenium: .002 mg., Zinc: .3 mg.

POTATO SALAD WITH AVOCADO DRESSING

preparation time: 30 min.
cooking time: 20 min.
chilling time: 1 hour

servings: 6

8 medium potatoes
1 small onion, diced (optional)
2 ribs celery, diced
1 cucumber, peeled and diced
1 cup raw or blanched diced broccoli
1 raw or blanched carrot, sliced
1 red or green bell pepper, diced

Avocado Dressing:
1 large, ripe avocado, peeled and
  pitted
1 cucumber, peeled and chopped
juice of 1 lemon
1 tsp. dill
2 Tbsp. soup stock or celery juice

❑ Steam the potatoes until tender. Peel and slice into 1-inch cubes. Combine the potatoes, onion, celery, diced cucumber, broccoli, carrot, and bell pepper in a large bowl.

❑ To make the dressing, combine the avocado, the chopped cucumber, lemon juice, dill, and stock or celery juice in a blender or food processor until smooth.

❑ Pour the dressing over the potato salad, and mix well. Chill and serve.

All information is per serving:

Calories: 278 (9% from protein, 17% from fat)
Protein: 6.6 gm., Fat: 5.5 gm., Linoleic Acid: .7 gm., Fiber: 7.8 gm.
Calcium: 55 mg., Sodium: 40 mg., Iron: 1.9 mg.
B-Carotene: 386 µg., Vitamin C: 72 mg., Vitamin E: 1.1 mg.
Selenium: .002 mg., Zinc: 1.1 mg.

HOLIDAY PEAR SALAD

preparation time: 15 min.

servings: 4

❑ Toss all the ingredients, except the endive or lettuce, just until coated with the juice. Arrange on a serving dish, and garnish the edges of the salad with endive or lettuce.

4 ripe pears, cored and diced
3 stalks celery, finely diced
1 small jicama, peeled and diced, or
  2 cups diced water chestnuts
1 cup sliced walnuts or pecans
1 cup pineapple juice
Belgium endive or romaine lettuce for garnish

All information is per serving:

Calories: 353 (9% from protein, 43% from fat)
Protein: 9 gm., Fat: 18.6 gm., Linoleic Acid: 10.7 gm., Fiber: 7.6 gm.
Calcium: 67 mg., Sodium: 38 mg., Iron: 1.9 mg.
B-Carotene: 14 µg., Vitamin C: 19 mg., Vitamin E: 1.5 mg.
Selenium: .007 mg., Zinc: 1.4 mg.

SUMMER SALAD SUPREME

preparation time: 25 min.

servings: 6

1 head of lettuce (can be 1/2 romaine and 1/2 red leaf), well washed and torn into pieces

4 carrots, finely shredded

1 jicama, coarsely shredded, or
   2 1/2 cups finely chopped water chestnuts

3 ribs celery, diced

1 red or green bell pepper, diced

1 cucumber, diced

4 oz. alfalfa sprouts

1 fresh tomato, sliced

2 mangoes, diced

1 pint red raspberries

5 ripe plums, pitted and diced

❑ Toss all the ingredients in a large bowl. The juices of the fruits will make a sweet "dressing" for this salad.

All information is per serving:

Calories: 138 (10% from protein, 7% from fat)

Protein: 3.9 gm., Fat: 1.2 gm., Linoleic Acid: .3 gm., Fiber: 7.0 gm.

Calcium: 70 mg., Sodium: 44 mg., Iron: 1.7 mg.

B-Carotene: 1672 µg., Vitamin C: 68 mg., Vitamin E: 2.0 mg.

Selenium: .002 mg., Zinc: .7 mg.

Rice-Tangerine Salad

preparation time: 30 min.
chilling time: 1 hour

servings: 6

❑ Combine all the ingredients in a large mixing bowl. Fluff with a fork, chill, and serve.

Hint: Honey tangelo, Mandarin orange, or Satsumi tangerines are the best.

6 cups cooked brown basmati rice
1 Tbsp. fresh basil, coarsely chopped
leaves from 1 bunch cilantro
2 cups fresh mung bean sprouts
3 tangerines, peeled, seeded, and separated into wedges

All information is per serving:

Calories: 247 (9% from protein, 6% from fat)
Protein: 5.9 gm., Fat: 1.8 gm., Linoleic Acid: .6 gm., Fiber: 4.6 gm.
Calcium: 32 mg., Sodium: 4.9 mg., Iron: 1.4 mg.
B-Carotene: .7 µg., Vitamin C: 18 mg., Vitamin E: 1.4 mg.
Selenium: .077 mg., Zinc: 1.5 mg.

TOMATO HERB SALAD

preparation time: 15 min.

servings: 4

1 cup arugula, chopped
1/2 cup fresh cilantro, minced
10 leaves fresh basil, minced
1 cucumber, thinly sliced
1 small jicama, peeled and diced, or
  2 cups diced water chestnuts
5 roma or Italian tomatoes, thinly
  sliced
2 cups small cherry tomatoes, cut in
  half
1 avocado, diced

❑ Toss all the ingredients together until well mixed.

All information is per serving:

Calories: 136 (10% from protein, 50% from fat)
Protein: 3.6 gm., Fat: 8.4 gm., Linoleic Acid: 1.1 gm., Fiber: 4.5 gm.
Calcium: 48 mg., Sodium: 29 mg., Iron: 1.8 mg.
B-Carotene: 243 µg., Vitamin C: 49 mg., Vitamin E: 1.8 mg.
Selenium: .002 mg., Zinc: .6 mg.

ASPARAGUS SALAD

preparation time: 20 min.
cooking time: 3 min.
chilling time: 1 hour

servings: 8

❑ Cut off the tough ends of the asparagus, and steam the tips 2-3 minutes, taking care not to overcook. When cool, cut into 1-inch pieces, and place in a large mixing bowl with the pumpkin seeds or almonds.

❑ Toss in the remaining ingredients. If the tomatoes are not too juicy, you may want to top the salad with 1/2 cup grapefruit juice or a light, healthful dressing. Chill and serve.

2 lbs. fresh asparagus
1/4 cup finely chopped raw pumpkin seeds or almonds

4 leaves romaine lettuce, torn into bite-size pieces
2 large tomatoes, diced
2 ribs celery, sliced
1 large head bok choy, sliced

All information is per serving:

Calories: 60 (29% from protein, 39% from fat)
Protein: 4.6 gm., Fat: 2.8 gm., Linoleic Acid: .9 gm., Fiber: 2.5 gm.
Calcium: 28 mg., Sodium: 43 mg., Iron: 1.8 mg.
B-Carotene: 163 µg., Vitamin C: 38 mg., Vitamin E: 2.6 mg.
Selenium: n/a, Zinc: 1.2 mg.

GREEN BEAN SALAD

preparation time: 30 min.
chilling time: 1 hour

servings: 4

7 cups (2 lbs.) fresh green beans, cut
   into 1-inch pieces and blanched
juice of 1 lemon
2 cloves garlic, minced, or 1/2 tsp.
   garlic powder
2 Tbsp. parsley flakes
1 tsp. basil

Optional ingredients:
1 medium fresh tomato, diced
1 red or green bell pepper, sliced and
   blanched
1 cup sliced, blanched mushrooms

❑ Combine all the ingredients and mix
well. Chill and serve.

All information is per serving:

Calories: 101 (18% from protein, 7% from fat)

Protein: 5.3 gm., Fat: .9 gm., Linoleic Acid: .2 gm., Fiber: 5.0 gm.

Calcium: 118 mg., Sodium: 13 mg., Iron: 3.8 mg.

B-Carotene: 193 µg., Vitamin C: 53 mg., Vitamin E: .3 mg.

Selenium: .005 mg., Zinc: 1.0 mg.

SWEET SCARLET SALAD DRESSING

preparation time: 25 min.

servings: 8 (makes1 1/2 cups)

❑ Steam the beets until tender, then cool. Place in a blender or food processor, and purée with a small amount of the juice. When smooth, add the remaining juice and the sage, and blend.

❑ Keep chilled.

2 large beets, diced (2 cups)
1/2 cup apple juice
1/2 cup celery juice or vegetable stock
1 tsp. sage

All information is per serving (1/3 cup):

Calories: 28 (10% from protein, 2% from fat)

Protein: .7 gm., Fat: .1 gm., Linoleic Acid: .02 gm., Fiber: 1.6 gm.

Calcium: 12 mg., Sodium: 39 mg., Iron: .5 mg.

B-Carotene: 2 μg., Vitamin C: 4 mg., Vitamin E: .2 mg.

Selenium: n/a, Zinc: .2 mg.

AVOCADO DRESSING

preparation time: 10 min.

servings: 2 (makes 1 cup)

1/2 tomato, diced
1 avocado, peeled and sliced
1/2 cup celery juice or water
8 basil leaves

❑ Place all the ingredients in a blender or food processor, and purée until smooth. Serve immediately.

Variation: Replace the basil with your favorite fresh herb (tarragon, cilantro, oregano, etc.).

All information is per serving (1/2 cup):

Calories: 170 (6% from protein, 74% from fat)

Protein: 2.6 gm., Fat: 15 gm., Linoleic Acid: 1.7 gm., Fiber: 4.4 gm.

Calcium: 43 mg., Sodium: 48 mg., Iron: 1.3 mg.

B-Carotene: 40 µg., Vitamin C: 16 mg., Vitamin E: 2.0 mg.

Selenium: .001 mg., Zinc: .5 mg.

KIWI DRESSING

preparation time: 10 min.

servings: 15 ounces

❑ Combine all the ingredients in a blender until thoroughly mixed.

3 kiwi, peeled
1 red or green bell pepper, cut into large chunks
1 rib celery, cut into large chunks
1/4 cup water
8 grapes

All information is per 2 tablespoon serving:

Calories: 32 (6% from protein, 6% from fat)
Protein: .6 gm., Fat: .2 gm., Linoleic Acid: .022 gm., Fiber: 1.7 gm.
Calcium: 15 mg., Sodium: 8 mg., Iron: .3 mg.
B-Carotene: 14 µg., Vitamin C: 49 mg., Vitamin E: .6 mg.
Selenium: n/a, Zinc: .1 mg.

69

CUCUMBER KIWI DRESSING

preparation time: 5 min.

servings: 4 (makes 1 cup)

1/2 cucumber, peeled and cut into
  large chunks
3 kiwis, peeled
2 Tbsp. water

❑ Combine all the ingredients in a blender until smooth.

All information is per serving (1/4 cup):

Calories: 40 (7% from protein, 6% from fat)

Protein: .8 gm., Fat: .3 gm., Linoleic Acid: .01 gm., Fiber: 1.9 gm.

Calcium: 20 mg., Sodium: 4 mg., Iron: .3 mg.

B-Carotene: 10 µg., Vitamin C: 58 mg., Vitamin E: .7 mg.

Selenium: n/a, Zinc: .2 mg.

VEGETABLE ENTREES

SKILLET RATATOUILLE

preparation time: 20 min.
cooking time: 60 min.

servings: 4

1 cup peeled, cubed eggplant
2 cups diced fresh tomatoes
1 clove garlic, minced (optional)
1 tsp. fresh oregano, or 1/2 tsp. dried
1 Tbsp. fresh basil, or 1/2 tsp. dried
1/2 cup vegetable stock or water

1 cup diced celery
2 cups diced red or green bell peppers
2/3 cup thinly sliced zucchini
2/3 cup thinly sliced mushrooms

Sauce:
1/2 cup tomato paste
1 cup apple juice
1 Tbsp. lemon juice
1 Tbsp. arrowroot

❑ In a large skillet, sauté the eggplant, tomatoes, garlic, and herbs in the vegetable stock or water until the eggplant just starts to soften (about 15 minutes). Add the remaining vegetables and cook until nearly done (about 20 minutes).

❑ Using a wire whisk, combine the sauce ingredients and pour over the vegetables. Mix well, cover, and cook until slightly thickened (about 25 minutes).

All information is per serving:

Calories: 145 (11% from protein, 7% from fat)
Protein: 4.6 gm., Fat: 1.2 gm., Linoleic .5 Acid: gm., Fiber: 5.6 gm.
Calcium: 57 mg., Sodium: 67 mg., Iron: 3.0 mg.
B-Carotene: 211 µg., Vitamin C: 175 mg., Vitamin E: 1.7 mg.
Selenium: .003 mg., Zinc: .8 mg.

MASHED POTATOES WITH A TWIST

preparation time: 20 min.
cooking time: 60 min.

servings: 5

❑ Bake the potatoes at 375° F for 60 minutes or until done. Cut the squash in half lengthwise, and remove the seeds. Place the squash face down on a baking tray, and bake at 375° F for 30 minutes or until tender. If using yams, bake them until done. If using eggplant, bake whole for 30 minutes until tender.

❑ Cut the potatoes open and scrape out the potato from the skin into a bowl; do the same with the squash. Mash together with a potato masher, or purée in a food processor, adding water if needed for smoothness. Serve topped with Roasted Carrot and Green Bean Purée (see p. 26) or Emerald Sauce (see p. 51).

Hints: Restuff the mixture into the potato skins, and bake at 425° F, and/or broil until browned on top. You can also steam these vegetables. If you dice them small, the cooking time is less.

4 large potatoes (russet, Yukon Gold, or red)

1 medium butternut or other hard squash, or 3 large yams, or 2 medium eggplants

All information is per serving:

Calories: 225 (8% from protein, 1% from fat)
Protein: 4.9 gm., Fat: .3 gm., Linoleic Acid: .07 gm., Fiber: 6.1 gm.
Calcium: 66 mg., Sodium: 18 mg., Iron: 2.9 mg.
B-Carotene: 0 µg., Vitamin C: 39 mg., Vitamin E: .2 mg.
Selenium: .002 mg., Zinc: .7 mg.

ITALIAN CAULIFLOWER MIX

preparation time: 15 min.
cooking time: 20 min.

servings: 6

1 head cauliflower, broken into florets

1 clove garlic, minced, or 1/2 tsp. garlic
powder
1/2 tsp. oregano
1/2 tsp. basil
1 yellow squash, cut into thin, 2-inch
strips
1 red bell pepper, sliced
3 tomatoes, cut into wedges
1/2 cup fresh or frozen green peas, or
snow peas or green beans

❑ Precook the cauliflower in a covered steamer basket until partially cooked but still firm. Save the steaming liquid.

❑ In a large, nonstick skillet, steam-fry the garlic, oregano, and basil for 1 minute with a few tablespoons of the steaming liquid.

❑ Add the cauliflower and a few more tablespoons of the reserved liquid, and stir-fry the cauliflower for 2 minutes.

❑ Add the squash, bell pepper, and more liquid if necessary. Stir-fry 2 more minutes; add the tomatoes and about 1/2 cup of the reserved liquid, cover, and steam for 2 minutes. Remove cover and add the peas.

❑ Continue to cook for another 3-4 minutes. Serve hot as an entree alone or as a side dish, or over pasta or rice.

All information is per serving:
Calories: 69 (23% from protein, 7% from fat)
Protein: 4.5 gm., Fat: .6 gm., Linoleic Acid: .2 gm., Fiber: 5.3 gm.
Calcium: 56 mg., Sodium: 17 mg., Iron: 1.4 mg.
B-Carotene: 84 µg., Vitamin C: 117 mg., Vitamin E: .3 mg.
Selenium: 0 mg., Zinc: .6 mg.

ST. PATTY'S POTATO CASSEROLE

preparation time: 30 min.
cooking time: 60 min.

servings: 6

❑ Braise the mushrooms, greens, and 1 leek bulb in the stock or water until tender. Blend in a food processor with the soymilk or rice milk, juice, sage, and thyme.

❑ When smooth, return to the pan, and whisk in the arrowroot. Heat until the sauce begins to thicken; cover and remove from the heat.

❑ Layer the potatoes, carrots, cabbage, celery, and remaining leek bulb in a 4-quart casserole dish. Pour the sauce over the layered potatoes and vegetables. Cover and bake at 350° F for 60 minutes, or until the potatoes are tender.

2 cups sliced mushrooms
1 cup finely chopped spinach or Swiss chard
1 leek bulb, sliced
1 cup soup stock or water
2 cups soymilk or Rice Milk (see p. 151)
1/2 cup apple juice
1/2 tsp. sage
1/2 tsp. thyme

1 Tbsp. arrowroot

4 medium red or Yukon Gold potatoes, sliced
2 medium carrots, peeled and sliced
1/2 head cabbage, sliced
4 stalks celery, chopped
1 leek bulb, sliced

All information is per serving:

Calories: 256 (11% from protein, 3% from fat)
Protein: 7.1 gm., Fat: .9 gm., Linoleic Acid: .2 gm., Fiber: 9.4 gm.
Calcium: 113 mg., Sodium: 119 mg., Iron: 4.2 mg.
B-Carotene: 774 µg., Vitamin C: 85 mg., Vitamin E: 1.3 mg.
Selenium: .029 mg., Zinc: 1.2 mg.

STUFFED SQUASH

preparation time: 60 min.
cooking time: 55 min.

servings: 6

1 large red bell pepper
7 ribs celery

6 large acorn squash

10 large button mushrooms
2 red or green bell peppers
1 bunch Swiss chard or kale
1 tsp. basil
1 tsp. oregano

❑ Juice the bell pepper and celery, and set aside. Reserve 1/2 cup of the juice for steaming the vegetables, and use the remainder for basting the Spicy Yam Chips on the next page.

❑ Preheat the oven to 375° F. Slice off the ends of the squash, then cut in half lengthwise and remove the seeds. Lay the squash face down on a baking sheet, and bake for 30 minutes or until tender. The surface of the cut squash that faces the baking sheet should caramelize and turn an attractive purplish brown.

❑ While the acorn squash is baking, steam the mushrooms and bell peppers in the 1/2 cup reserved celery-red pepper juice until slightly tender.

❑ Add the chard or kale, and continue to steam until all the vegetables are tender but still firm and bright in color. Stir in the herbs.

❑ When the squash is done, spoon the vegetables into the seed cavity, and serve on a plate surrounded by Spicy Yam Chips (see facing page).

All information is per serving:

Calories: 143 (9% from protein, 3% from fat)
Protein: 3.8 gm., Fat: .6 gm., Linoleic Acid: .15 gm., Fiber: 6.4 gm.
Calcium: 49 mg., Sodium: 51 mg., Iron: 1.6 mg.
B-Carotene: 85 µg., Vitamin C: 63 mg., Vitamin E: 9 mg.
Selenium: .004 mg., Zinc: .7 mg.

SPICY YAM CHIPS

preparation time: 20 min.
cooking time: 25 min.

servings: 6

☐ Preheat the oven to 425° F. Peel the yams and cut lengthwise into 1/4-inch thick slices. Cover the bottom of a baking pan (you may need two) with some of the pepper/celery juice.

☐ Arrange the yams in the bottom of the pan, and add the rest of the juice to not quite cover.

☐ Mix the spices together in a bowl, and sprinkle evenly over the yams. Bake for 25 minutes or until just tender. Broil each tray until the tops of the yams are slightly brown.

5 yams
2 cups celery-red pepper juice (see Stuffed Squash recipe on facing page)

1 Tbsp. garlic powder
1 Tbsp. cumin
1 Tbsp. oregano

All information is per serving:

Calories: 138 (9% from protein, 3% from fat)
Protein: 3.6 gm., Fat: .5 gm., Linoleic Acid: .1 gm., Fiber: 6.1 gm.
Calcium: 137 mg., Sodium: 103 mg., Iron: 3.2 mg.
B-Carotene: 110 µg., Vitamin C: 53 mg., Vitamin E: 1.0 mg.
Selenium: .015 mg., Zinc: .6 mg.

STUFFED ZUCCHINI

preparation time: 55 min.
cooking time: 25 min.

servings: 6

6 medium zucchini
4 1/2 cups soup stock
1 1/2 cups uncooked brown rice
1/4 cup uncooked millet
1/4 cup uncooked wild rice

1 leek bulb, chopped, or 2 tsp. onion powder
4 cups sliced mushrooms
1 tsp. thyme
1 tsp. sage

2 cups Vegetable Marinara Sauce (see p. 47) or your favorite tomato sauce

❑ Steam or bake the whole zucchini until slightly tender, then allow to cool. Bring the stock to a boil, and add the rice, millet, and wild rice.

❑ Meanwhile, in a 2-quart skillet, steam-fry the leek, mushrooms, thyme, and sage in 1/2 cup of water, until the leeks and mushrooms are tender. Cover and simmer on low for 40 minutes.

❑ Remove the cooked rice from the heat, and let stand for 10 minutes, covered. Slice the zucchini lengthwise; scoop out the seeds and place the pulp in a large bowl. Stir in the vegetable mixture, and gently toss in the rice.

❑ Preheat the oven to 350° F. Spoon the filling into the zucchini halves. Place the halves in a casserole pan with 2-3 tablespoons of water on the bottom.

❑ Cover and bake for 25 minutes. Top with Vegetable Marinara Sauce, and serve.

All information is per serving:

Calories: 291 (12% from protein, 7% from fat)
Protein: 9.0 gm., Fat: 2.1 gm., Linoleic Acid: .8 gm., Fiber: 6.7 gm.
Calcium: 56 mg., Sodium: 39 mg., Iron: 3.2 mg.
B-Carotene: 98 µg., Vitamin C: 20 mg., Vitamin E: 1.6 mg.
Selenium: .02 mg., Zinc: 2.2 mg.

BUTTERNUT CORN HOTPOT

preparation time: 30 min.
cooking time: 20 min.

servings: 6

❑ Steam the squash, carrots, peas or beans, and ears of corn until tender (about 10 minutes).

❑ Braise the mushrooms and sage in 2 tablespoons of water for 5 minutes. Remove from the heat.

❑ Cut off the corn kernels as close to the cob as possible. Mix the corn kernels with the rosemary and sage, and set aside.

❑ Mix the remaining vegetables with the thyme, and spread evenly in an 8-quart casserole dish.

❑ Top with the corn and then the steamed mushrooms. Cover and bake at 350° F for 20 minutes until heated through.

4 cups butternut squash, peeled, deseeded, and cut in 1/2-inch cubes (1 1/2 lbs.)

3 medium carrots, cleaned and sliced in 1/2-inch thick rounds

2 cups fresh peas or fresh green beans, cut in 1-inch lengths

4 ears young sweet corn

2 cups diced fresh mushrooms

1 tsp. rosemary
1 tsp. ground sage

1 tsp. thyme

All information is per serving:

Calories: 141 (16% from protein, 3% from fat)
Protein: 6.5 gm., Fat: .6 gm., Linoleic Acid: .1 gm., Fiber: 5.0 gm.
Calcium: 82 mg., Sodium: 22 mg., Iron: 2.1 mg.
B-Carotene: 1049 µg., Vitamin C: 38 mg., Vitamin E: .5 mg.
Selenium: .005 mg., Zinc: 1.1 mg.

HOME FRIES

preparation time: 15 min.
cooking time: 30 min.

servings: 6

6 cups potatoes, cleaned and diced
1 cup stock or celery juice

1/2 cup stock or water
3 cups sliced mushrooms
1 red or green bell pepper, diced
1 small yellow onion, diced, or 1/2 cup
  chopped green onions
2 Tbsp. parsley

❑ Steam the potatoes in 1 cup stock or celery juice until tender (about 20-30 minutes).

❑ Steam the remaining ingredients in 1/2 cup stock or water until tender (about 10 minutes).

❑ Stir in the potatoes, heat through, and serve hot. This dish is great served with Homemade Ketchup (see p. 49), salsa, or as is.

All information is per serving:

Calories: 236 (10% from protein, 2% from fat)
Protein: 6.3 gm., Fat: .5 gm., Linoleic Acid: .2 gm., Fiber: 5.0 gm.
Calcium: 39 mg., Sodium: 17 mg., Iron: 3.0 mg.
B-Carotene: 74 µg., Vitamin C: 106 mg., Vitamin E: .1 mg.
Selenium: .005 mg., Zinc: 1.2 mg.

ARTICHOKES WITH FRESH TOMATO SAUCE

preparation time: 30 min.
cooking time: 30 min.

servings: 4

□ Rinse the artichokes. Cut off the stems close to the base, and cut off the tops (approximately 1 inch). Steam the artichokes in a large pot by bringing 2 inches of water to a boil and adding the lemon slices and artichokes.

□ Cover, reduce the heat to medium-low, and simmer 25 to 30 minutes, or until the artichokes are tender. Remove the artichokes from the pot, and turn them upside down on a platter to drain.

□ To make the sauce, place the onions, garlic, and a few tablespoons of water in a large skillet, and steam-fry until soft. Stir in the chopped tomatoes and the remaining ingredients. Simmer over low heat for 15 minutes, stirring occasionally.

□ Place the artichokes on individual serving dishes, and spoon the tomato sauce around them. To eat, pull off a leaf, dip into the sauce, and draw the fleshy portion out between the teeth. Discard the remainder of the leaf.

□ When you reach the center, remove the pointy inner leaves, and, using a knife or the edge of a spoon, scrape out the "hairs." Dip the artichoke bottom into the sauce, and enjoy!

4 medium artichokes
1 lemon, sliced

2 Tbsp. chopped onions (optional)
1 clove garlic, minced, or 1 tsp. garlic powder
6 cups chopped tomatoes
1/2 cup chopped parsley
1/4 cup lemon juice
1 tsp. basil
1/2 tsp. rosemary

All information is per serving:

Calories: 173 (17% from protein, 8% from fat)
Protein: 8.6 gm., Fat: 1.8 gm., Linoleic Acid: .7 gm., Fiber: 7.4 gm.
Calcium: 103 mg., Sodium: 159 mg., Iron: 4.3 mg.
B-Carotene: 423 µg., Vitamin C: 119 mg., Vitamin E: 1.6 mg.
Selenium: .002 mg., Zinc: 1.1 mg.

SHEPHERD'S PIE

preparation time: 30 min.
cooking time: 60 min.

servings: 8

10 potatoes, peeled and steamed (save the water)
1 small yam, peeled and steamed
8 cups bite-sized vegetables, such as: carrots, celery, broccoli, cauliflower, red or green bell peppers, corn, mushrooms, peas, zucchini, or yellow squash
3 cups favorite gravy or sauce
chopped fresh parsley for a garnish

❑ In a food processor, purée the potatoes and yam using the water from steaming if needed.

❑ Preheat the oven to 350° F. Place the bite-sized vegetable pieces in a 4-quart casserole dish, and top with the 3 cups of gravy.

❑ Spread the puréed potatoes over the top all the way to the edge, to seal in moisture.

❑ Sprinkle the chopped parsley over the potatoes, and bake for 60 minutes, or until the vegetables are tender. Serve hot!

All information is per serving:

Calories: 398 (11% from protein, 2% from fat)
Protein: 11 gm., Fat: 1.0 gm., Linoleic Acid: .2 gm., Fiber: 11.8 gm.
Calcium: 68 mg., Sodium: 93 mg., Iron: 4.8 mg.
B-Carotene: 766 µg., Vitamin C: 90 mg., Vitamin E: 2.4 mg.
Selenium: .004 mg., Zinc: 1.3 mg.

SPAGHETTI SQUASH "PASTA"

preparation time: 15 min.
cooking time: 60 min.

servings: 5

❑ With a large knife, cut the squash in half lengthwise. Remove and discard the seeds. Place the squash cut side down on a baking sheet, and bake at 350° F for 60 minutes, or until just tender. Be careful not to overcook.

❑ Combine all the sauce ingredients in a 4-quart saucepan, and simmer at least 30 minutes.

❑ When the spaghetti squash is done, pull the squash strands from the skin using a fork. Place about 1 cup of "spaghetti" on each plate, and top with 1/2 cup of the warm sauce. Serve immediately.

Variation: Use the Vegetable Marinara Sauce on p. 47 or the Rich Red Sauce on p. 45.

1 large spaghetti squash (approximately 5 lbs.)

Sauce:
18 oz. tomato paste
4 cups water
1 clove garlic, minced (optional)
1 1/2 tsp. oregano
1 1/2 tsp. basil

All information is per serving:

Calories: 210 (10% from protein, 4% from fat)
Protein: 8 gm., Fat: 14 gm., Linoleic Acid: 14 gm., Fiber: 12 gm.
Calcium: 242 mg., Sodium: 91 mg., Iron: 6.2 mg.
B-Carotene: n/a, Vitamin C: 112 mg., Vitamin E: .5 mg.
Selenium: .006 mg., Zinc: 1.5 mg.

ROOT-A-BAKA

preparation time: 25 min.
cooking time: 60 min.

servings: 8

2 Yukon Gold potatoes
6 russet potatoes, peeled
2 large carrots, peeled
3 medium beets, peeled
3 medium turnips
2 medium parsnips
2 medium yams
3 1/2 cups celery juice or stock

❑ Preheat the oven to 350° F. Slice all the vegetables into rounds 1/4-inch thick. Layer in a 4-quart casserole dish.

❑ Pour the juice or stock over the vegetables, and cover. Bake for 60 minutes.

All information is per serving:

Calories: 258 (8% from protein, 1% from fat)
Protein: 5.6 gm., Fat: 5.6 gm., Linoleic Acid: .1 gm., Fiber: 7.9 gm.
Calcium: 44 mg., Sodium: 56 mg., Iron: 3.2 mg.
B-Carotene: 657 µg., Vitamin C: 35 mg., Vitamin E: 1.0 mg.
Selenium: .002 mg., Zinc: .9 mg.

SCALLOPED POTATOES

preparation time: 25 min.
cooking time: 60 min.

servings: 4

1 cup water
1/2 cup apple juice
4 cups chopped Swiss chard or kale

2 cups soymilk or Rice Milk
  (see p. 151)
1/4 leek, sliced
1/2 tsp. thyme
1 tsp. arrowroot

4 medium potatoes, sliced
2 cups sliced mushrooms
1 cup sliced onion (optional)

❑ Heat the water and apple juice in a nonstick pan, and steam-fry the chard until soft. Purée the greens in a food processor until smooth, then return to the pan.

❑ In a blender, purée the soymilk or rice milk, leek, thyme, and arrowroot. Add to the greens and heat on low until a thick gravy is formed.

❑ Preheat the oven to 350° F. Layer the potatoes, mushrooms, and onion in a casserole dish. Pour the gravy over the layered potatoes and mushrooms. Cover and bake for 60 minutes, or until the potatoes are tender.

Hint: If leftover split pea or yam soup is available, it may be used in place of the gravy.

All information is per serving:

Calories: 341 (11% from protein, 2% from fat)
Protein: 10.0 gm., Fat: 1.0 gm., Linoleic Acid: .3 gm., Fiber: 10.5 gm.
Calcium: 139.4 mg., Sodium: 335 mg., Iron: 7.8 mg.
B-Carotene: 547 µg., Vitamin C: 60 mg., Vitamin E: 3.2 mg.
Selenium: .095 mg., Zinc: 1.8 mg.

REBAKED POTATOES

preparation time: 30 min.
cooking time: 75 min.

servings: 6

6 large russet potatoes

1/2 cup finely chopped chives, or 2 tsp. dried

1 tsp. onion powder (optional)
1/2 cup minced fresh parsley, or 4 tsp. dried

2 cooked medium yams

❑ Bake the potatoes for 1 hour at 375° F. While the potatoes are still warm, slice them lengthwise and scoop the potatoes from the skins.

❑ Place the skins in a shallow baking dish, and put the potato in a large mixing bowl. Mash the potato with the chives, onion powder, parsley, and yams.

❑ Spoon the mixture back into the skins. Broil until the tops start to brown. Serve hot or cold.

All information is per serving:

Calories: 264 (8% from protein, 1% from fat)
Protein: 5.6 gm., Fat: .3 gm., Linoleic Acid: .1 gm., Fiber: 6.2 gm.
Calcium: 43 mg., Sodium: 23 mg., Iron: 3.3 mg.
B-Carotene: 829 µg., Vitamin C: 45 mg., Vitamin E: 1.9 mg.
Selenium: .001 mg., Zinc: .9 mg.

RATATOUILLE

preparation time: 30 min.
cooking time: 45 min.

servings: 6

❑ In a 3-quart skillet, steam-fry the bell pepper strips and seasonings in 3/4 cup stock, celery juice, or water until soft.

❑ Add the eggplants, carrots, zucchini, mushrooms, tomatoes, and spinach. Stir well and transfer to 4-quart casserole dish.

❑ Preheat the oven to 350° F. Fill the casserole with liquid to two-thirds full. Cover and bake covered for 30 minutes.

❑ Whisk together the apple juice and arrowroot. Stir into the vegetables and bake an additional 15 minutes. Serve hot over rice or other grain.

2 red or green bell peppers, sliced into thin strips
2 bay leaves
2 tsp. basil
2 tsp. oregano
1 1/2 tsp. garlic powder
soup stock, celery juice, or water

2 small eggplants, diced into 1-inch cubes
3 carrots, sliced
2 zucchini, sliced
6 mushrooms, sliced
3 tomatoes, diced
1 bunch spinach or chard, washed well and coarsely chopped

1/2 cup apple juice
2 Tbsp. arrowroot

All information is per serving:

Calories: 83 (10% from protein, 7% from fat)
Protein: 2.4 gm., Fat: .7 gm., Linoleic Acid: .2 gm., Fiber: 4.6 gm.
Calcium: 52 mg., Sodium: 29.5 mg., Iron: 1.7 mg.
B-Carotene: 1168 µg., Vitamin C: 42 mg., Vitamin E: .8 mg.
Selenium: .002 mg., Zinc: .4 mg.

GRAIN ENTREES

POLENTA SQUARES

preparation time: 20 min.
cooking time: 1 hour, 15 min.

servings: 4

2 1/2 cups soup stock or water, or celery/pepper/tomato juice
1/2 cup apple juice
6 oz. tomato paste
1 leek, finely chopped, or 2 tsp. onion powder
1 rib celery, finely chopped

Pizza Style:
1/2 red or green pepper, diced
1 Tbsp. basil
1/2 Tbsp. garlic powder
1/2 Tbsp. oregano
1/2 cup chopped mushrooms
1/2 cup diced fresh tomatoes

Tamale Style:
1/2 red or green bell pepper, diced
1 Tbsp. cumin
1/2 Tbsp. garlic powder
1/2 Tbsp. cilantro
1/2 cup diced fresh tomatoes

1 cup white or yellow cornmeal

❑ In an 8-quart saucepan, bring the stock or water to a boil, and add the apple juice, tomato paste, leek, celery, and the flavorings of your choice. Lower to medium-low heat, and simmer for 10 minutes.

❑ Preheat the oven to 350° F. Add the cornmeal, stirring constantly, and cook for 2-3 minutes until most of the liquid is absorbed. Spread into a nonstick baking pan with a 1/2-inch edge, and bake for 25 minutes. Let cool completely so that the polenta will firm up. Reheat quickly when ready to top.

❑ For Pizza-style polenta, top with Vegetable Marinara Sauce (see p. 47) and sautéed vegetables.

❑ For Tamale-style polenta, top with cooked beans, rice, lettuce, and salsa or guacamole. Slice into squares and serve.

All information is per serving:

Calories: 241.8 (11% from protein, 5% from fat)
Protein: 7.2 gm., Fat: 1.376 gm., Linoleic Acid: .5 gm., Fiber: 6.8 gm.
Calcium: 69 mg., Sodium: 64 mg., Iron: 3.9 mg.
B-Carotene: 41 µg., Vitamin C: 66 mg., Vitamin E: .8 mg.
Selenium: .004 mg., Zinc: 1.0 mg.

MILLET MASHED POTATOES

preparation time: 15 min.
cooking time: 30 min.

servings: 7

❑ In an 8-quart soup pot, bring the stock and juice to a boil. Meanwhile, toast the millet over medium heat in a nonstick pan until brown.

❑ Add all the ingredients, including the millet, to the boiling liquid. Cover and simmer for 25-30 minutes or until soft.

❑ Blend with a hand mixer or potato masher until well mixed. Serve with gravy or Emerald Sauce (see p. 51).

8 cups soup stock or water, or 7 cups soup stock or water and 1 cup celery juice
2 cups uncooked millet
6 russet potatoes, peeled and cubed
2 cups finely chopped cauliflower

All information is per serving:

Calories: 352 (11% from protein, 7% from fat)
Protein: 9.7 gm., Fat: 2.7 gm., Linoleic Acid: 1.3 gm., Fiber: 12 gm.
Calcium: 32 mg., Sodium: 42 mg., Iron: 2.4 mg.
B-Carotene: 3.0 µg., Vitamin C: 35 mg., Vitamin E: .2 mg.
Selenium: .001 mg., Zinc: 1.5 mg.

MILLET MAGIC

preparation time: 15 min.
cooking time: 60 min.

servings: 6

7 cups soup stock or water, or 4 cups water and 3 cups carrot juice
3 carrots, finely chopped
2 yams, peeled and finely chopped (4 cups)
4 cups sliced mushrooms
1 bunch green onions, sliced
1 Tbsp. parsley
1 tsp. sage
1 tsp. rosemary
1 tsp. thyme

1 cup uncooked millet
1 cup uncooked wild rice

❑ In a 4-quart saucepan, bring the stock or water to a boil. Add the carrots, yams, mushrooms, onions, and seasonings.

❑ Return to a boil and simmer for 10 minutes.

❑ Add the millet and wild rice, cover, and cook on medium heat for about 45 minutes, or until all the liquid is absorbed.

❑ Serve as is or top with a vegetable sauce.

All information is per serving:

Calories: 352 (12% from protein, 6% from fat)
Protein: 10.9 gm., Fat: 2.3 gm., Linoleic Acid: 1.0 gm., Fiber: 10.8 gm.
Calcium: 70 mg., Sodium: 63 mg., Iron: 3.6 mg.
B-Carotene: 4922 µg., Vitamin C: 23 mg., Vitamin E: 2.4 mg.
Selenium: .008 mg., Zinc: 3.0 mg.

PHONY MACARONI AND CHEESE

preparation time: 10 min.
cooking time: 30 min.

servings: 8

❑ Preheat the oven to 375° F.

❑ Place the corn elbows, the stock or juice, and water into a 4-quart baking dish. Stir, cover, and bake for 10 minutes.

❑ Top evenly with the squash. Cover and bake for 20 minutes more. Remove from the oven and serve.

6 cups corn elbow pasta
3 cups vegetable stock, or juice made from 2 red bell peppers, 6 ribs celery, and 2 cored apples
2 cups water

6 cups shredded butternut squash

All information is per serving:

Calories: 443 (7% from protein, 5% from fat)
Protein: 8.4 gm., Fat: 2.8 gm., Linoleic Acid: .7 gm., Fiber: 12.3 gm.
Calcium: 104 mg., Sodium: 68 mg., Iron: 3.1 mg.
B-Carotene: 73 µg., Vitamin C: 68 mg., Vitamin E: 2.4 mg.
Selenium: .002 mg., Zinc: 1.8 mg.

ITALIAN VEGETABLE STEW

preparation time: 35 min.
cooking time: 45 min.

servings: 12

12 cups soup stock or water
6 cups peeled, chopped potatoes
2 cups sliced carrots
3 cups sliced celery
2 leeks, sliced

3 cups sliced green beans (1-inch
  pieces)
2 cups sliced mushrooms
2 cups chopped zucchini

2 cups chopped cauliflower
3 cups fresh corn kernels
2 Tbsp. Italian seasonings, or 1 Tbsp.
  basil, 1/2 Tbsp. oregano, and 1/2
  Tbsp. thyme

6 oz. tomato paste
1/2 cup apple juice
3 cups corn elbow pasta, cooked just
  prior to using

❑ In an 8-quart soup pot, bring the stock or water to a boil. Add the potatoes, carrots, celery, and leeks, and cook over medium-high heat for 15 minutes.

❑ Add the green beans, mushrooms, and zucchini, and cook for 10 more minutes.

❑ Add the cauliflower, corn, and seasonings, and cook for 5 more minutes.

❑ Add the tomato paste and apple juice, stir well, then let simmer for 5-10 minutes on low heat. Gently stir in the cooked pasta, and remove from the heat. Serve immediately.

All information is per serving:

Calories: 287 (10% from protein, 4% from fat)
Protein: 7.5 gm., Fat: 1.4 gm., Linoleic Acid: .5 gm., Fiber: 6.3 gm.
Calcium: 74 mg., Sodium: 75 mg., Iron: 2.7 mg.
B-Carotene: 1024 µg., Vitamin C: 44 mg., Vitamin E: .8 mg.
Selenium: .004 mg., Zinc: 1.5 mg.

CHEESE-FREE EGGPLANT PARMESAN

preparation time: 15 min.
cooking time: 35 min.

servings: 4

❑ Coat the bottom of a 4-quart baking dish with a thin layer of Vegetable Marinara Sauce.

❑ Dip the eggplant slices in the ground oats, and arrange in the baking dish.

❑ Preheat the oven to 375° F. Layer the tomatoes, celery, bell pepper, and ground oats, then repeat for the second layer. Cover evenly with the remaining Vegetable Marinara Sauce.

❑ Cover and bake for 30 minutes. Remove the cover and broil for 5 minutes.

3 cups Vegetable Marinara Sauce (see p. 47)

1 medium eggplant, peeled and sliced into 1-inch rounds

1 cup oats, ground in a blender or food processor

2 medium tomatoes, thinly sliced

2 ribs celery, diced

1 large red or green bell pepper, thinly sliced

All information is per serving:

Calories: 246 (15% from protein, 12% from fat)

Protein: 10.0 gm., Fat: 3.6 gm., Linoleic Acid: 1.3 gm., Fiber: 11.7 gm.

Calcium: 64 mg., Sodium: 50 mg., Iron: 4.0 mg.

B-Carotene: 122 µg., Vitamin C: 51mg., Vitamin E: 1.1 mg.

Selenium: .013 mg., Zinc: 2.2 mg.

CORN PASTA

preparation time: 5 min.
cooking time: 5 min.

servings: 2

4 cups water or stock
2 cups corn elbows

❑ In a 4-quart saucepan, bring the water or stock to a boil. Add the pasta and stir frequently for 3 to 5 minutes, making sure not to overcook.

❑ Drain and rinse with hot water. Serve with a sauce or gravy.

Hint: Corn pasta is most easily prepared in elbow form as it tends to cook quickly and stick together. Top elbows with a sauce immediately to prevent from sticking.

All information is per serving:

Calories: 352 (8% from protein, 5% from fat)

Protein: 7.4 gm., Fat: 2.0 gm., Linoleic Acid: .9 gm., Fiber: 3.5 gm.

Calcium: 4 mg., Sodium: 2 mg., Iron: .7 mg.

B-Carotene: 15 µg., Vitamin C: n/a, Vitamin E: 1.0 mg.

Selenium: n/a, Zinc: 1.8 mg.

MILLET BURGERS

preparation time: 25 min.
cooking time: 50 min.

servings: 12

☐ In a 4-quart saucepan, bring the millet, liquid, and vegetables to a boil. Cover and simmer on low heat for 30 minutes, or until all the liquid has been absorbed. Allow to cool.

☐ In a large bowl, mix the millet mixture, bread crumbs, and seasonings. With wet hands, form the mixture into 12 balls. (Wet your hands to keep the millet from sticking.)

☐ Preheat the oven to 350° F. Press each ball into a patty, and place on a nonstick baking sheet. Bake for 10 minutes on each side.

2 cups plus 2 Tbsp. millet
4 1/2 cups stock, water, or carrot-celery juice
1 1/2 cups finely chopped vegetables (carrots, celery, etc.)

1 cup wheat-free bread crumbs
1 Tbsp. fresh summer savory, or 1/2 Tbsp. dried savory
1 Tbsp. onion powder
1 Tbsp. dried chives

All information is per serving (1 patty):

Calories: 177 (12% from protein, 10% from fat)
Protein: 5.2 gm., Fat: 2.0 gm., Linoleic Acid: .8 gm., Fiber: 5.6 gm.
Calcium: 41 mg., Sodium: 89 mg., Iron: 1.9 mg.
B-Carotene: 792 µg., Vitamin C: 2.9 mg., Vitamin E: .1 mg.
Selenium: n/a, Zinc: .8 mg.

POLENTA WITH SUN-DRIED TOMATOES

preparation time: 20 min.
cooking time: 25 min.

servings: 6

5 cups water
1 cup whole sun-dried tomatoes
2 tomatoes, diced
2 cups cleaned, sliced crimini or
  button mushrooms
1 red or green bell pepper, diced
2 tsp. oregano
2 tsp. basil
2 tsp. garlic powder

2 cups white or yellow cornmeal

1 bunch spinach, well washed, stems
  removed, and chopped

❑ In a 4-quart saucepan, bring the water, vegetables (except the spinach), and herbs to a boil.

❑ Add the cornmeal slowly while stirring, and continue to stir while cooking for 10 minutes. Stir in the spinach.

❑ Preheat the oven to 375° F. Pour the polenta into a baking dish large enough so that the polenta is about 2 inches thick. Cover and bake until firm, about 25 minutes. When done, let it cool slightly to thicken before slicing.

Variation: Decorate the polenta before baking with sliced tomatoes and fresh basil leaves.

All information is per serving:

Calories: 214 (13% from protein, 5% from fat)

Protein: 7.1 gm., Fat: 1.3 gm., Linoleic Acid: .5 gm., Fiber: 5.9 gm.

Calcium: 79 mg., Sodium: 393 mg., Iron: 2.9 mg.

B-Carotene: 255 µg., Vitamin C: n/a, Vitamin E: 1.0 mg.

Selenium: .002 mg., Zinc: 1.3 mg.

ENCHILADAS

preparation time: 45 min.
cooking time: 20 min.

servings: 12

❑ Heat the tortillas in a toaster oven or in a nonstick skillet until soft enough to roll without cracking. Place enough Enchilada Sauce in the bottom of a rectangular baking pan just to coat.

❑ Dip each tortilla in the remaining Enchilada Sauce, coating both sides, and place the tortilla on a plate. Spoon on 3-5 Tbsp. of rice and/or beans, roll up, and place in the prepared pan with the seams down. Continue to place the remaining filled tortillas one next to another in the pan.

❑ Preheat the oven to 350° F. Lightly coat the top of the enchiladas with the sauce (keeping any remaining sauce warm to serve over the baked enchiladas). Bake for 20 minutes.

Variation: Serve topped with guacamole or avocado slices. Alternative fillings could be mashed yams, mashed potatoes, or Killer Black Beans (see p. 112).

12 corn tortillas
8 cups Enchilada Sauce (see p. 50)
4 cups cooked rice and/or beans

All information is per serving (1 enchilada):

Calories: 175 (11% from protein, 9% from fat)
Protein: 5.0 gm., Fat: 1.7 gm., Linoleic Acid: .6 gm., Fiber: 3.4 gm.
Calcium: 78 mg., Sodium: 85 mg., Iron: 2.4 mg.
B-Carotene: 1.8 µg., Vitamin C: 22 mg., Vitamin E: .5 mg.
Selenium: .026 mg., Zinc: 1.1 mg.

VEGETABLE QUINOA

preparation time: 10 min.
cooking time: 35 min.

servings: 4

2 cups uncooked quinoa, rinsed
3 cups water
1 carrot, diced
1 red or green bell pepper, diced
1 cup well washed and torn spinach

❑ Rinse the quinoa, then bring 3 cups of water to a boil. Add the vegetables, then the quinoa.

❑ Return to a boil, then cook over low heat for 30 minutes. Remove from the heat and let set covered for 5 minutes. Remove the lid and fluff with a fork.

All information is per serving:

Calories: 334 (14% from protein, 13% from fat)
Protein: 11.9 gm., Fat: 5.0 gm., Linoleic Acid: 1.9 gm., Fiber: 5.5 gm.
Calcium: 75 mg., Sodium: 40.1 mg., Iron: 8.4 mg.
B-Carotene: 610 µg., Vitamin C: 22 mg., Vitamin E: .5 mg.
Selenium: .001 mg., Zinc: 3.0 mg.

BARLEY BURGERS

preparation time: 10 min.
cooking time: 25 min.

servings: 9

❑ Blend all the ingredients in a food processor until smooth and the consistency is that of a sticky dough. Shape into 9 patties. (Wet your hands first to avoid sticking.)

❑ Preheat the oven to 350° F. Place on a nonstick baking sheet, and bake for 10 minutes on each side. Then broil for 1 minute on each side, or until golden brown.

4 cups cooked barley
4 tsp. onion powder, or 1 medium onion, chopped
1/2 cup grated raw potato
1/2 cup minced green pepper
1/2 tsp. thyme

All information is per serving (1 patty):

Calories: 103 (8% from protein, 3% from fat)
Protein: 2.1 gm., Fat: .4 gm., Linoleic Acid: .2 gm., Fiber: 4.4 gm.
Calcium: 15 mg., Sodium: 4 mg., Iron: 1.2 mg.
B-Carotene: 7 µg., Vitamin C: 14 mg., Vitamin E: 1.9 mg.
Selenium: .046 mg., Zinc: .7 mg.

POLENTA VEGETABLE CASSEROLE

preparation time: 30 min.
cooking time: 25 min.

servings: 8

6 cups soup stock or water, or combine
  2 1/2 cups carrot-celery juice and
  3 1/2 cups water
8 cups chopped vegetables (zucchini,
  mushrooms, red or green bell
  peppers, spinach, leeks, corn,
  tomatoes, etc.)
1 Tbsp. oregano
1 Tbsp. basil
1 Tbsp. garlic powder

2 cups white or yellow cornmeal

❑ In an 8-quart soup pot, bring the stock or water to a boil, and stir in all the vegetables and seasonings. Simmer for 15 minutes until the vegetables are tender.

❑ Preheat the oven to 350° F. Slowly add the cornmeal to the soup pot, and stir constantly on low heat for 5 more minutes, until the cornmeal begins to thicken.

❑ Remove from the heat, spoon into a 4-quart casserole dish, and bake uncovered for 20-25 minutes. Serve hot and top with Emerald Sauce (see p. 51), Vegetable Marinara Sauce (see p. 47), or gravy.

All information is per serving:

Calories: 211 (10% from protein, 6% from fat)
Protein: 5.8 gm., Fat: 1.5 gm., Linoleic Acid: .6 gm., Fiber: 8.8 gm.
Calcium: 59 mg., Sodium: 47 mg., Iron: 2.8 mg.
B-Carotene: 1997 µg., Vitamin C: 14 mg., Vitamin E: .4 mg.
Selenium: .005 mg., Zinc: 1.2 mg.

LASAGNE

preparation time: 45 min.
cooking time: 60-90 min.

servings: 8

☐ In a 4-quart baking dish, layer 2 cups Vegetable Marinara Sauce, 2 cups corn elbows, the eggplant or zucchini, an additional 2 cups Vegetable Marinara Sauce, 2 more cups corn elbows, the kale or spinach, the bell pepper, 2 cups Vegetable Marinara Sauce, the remaining corn elbows, and 2 more cups Vegetable Marinara Sauce.

☐ Preheat the oven to 350° F. Add the stock or thinned Vegetable Marinara Sauce around the edges of the baking dish. Cover and bake for 30 minutes.

☐ Test the lasagne with a fork for tenderness and bake longer if needed.

8 cups Vegetable Marinara Sauce (see p. 47)

6 cups uncooked corn elbows

1 small eggplant or 3 medium zucchini, sliced

1 large bunch fresh spinach or kale, well washed and stems removed

1 red or green bell pepper, thinly sliced

1 medium yellow onion, sliced, or 2 leek bulbs, sliced

1 cup stock or thinned Vegetable Marinara Sauce

Variation: Replace the spinach layer by blending the spinach or kale, 2 cups crumbled medium-firm tofu, and 1/2 cup chopped yellow onion in a food processor. Let stand for 30 minutes.

All information is per serving:

Calories: 408 (12% from protein, 6% from fat)

Protein: 11.9 gm., Fat: 2.6 gm., Linoleic Acid: .56 gm., Fiber: 10.6 gm.

Calcium: 87 mg., Sodium: 87 mg., Iron: 4.0 mg.

B-Carotene: 211 µg., Vitamin C: 58 mg., Vitamin E: 0.75 mg.

Selenium: 5.3 mg., Zinc: 2.4 mg.

SPINACH RICE

preparation time: 30 min.
cooking time: 60 min.

servings: 7

2 1/2 cups uncooked basmati rice
1/4 cup uncooked wild rice or japonica rice
1 tsp. thyme
1 tsp. sage
1 tsp. garlic powder

1 large bunch spinach, well washed
1 cup water

6 large button mushrooms, sliced
1 red or green bell pepper, diced

5 cups soup stock or water

❑ Dry roast the basmati rice, wild rice, and herbs in a large sauté pan over high heat, stirring constantly.

❑ Blend the spinach in a food processor with 1 cup of water.

❑ Reduce the heat under the sauté pan to medium-low, and add the spinach, mushrooms, and bell pepper. Steam-fry for 5 minutes, stirring constantly.

❑ Preheat the oven to 350° F. Put the rice mixture into a 9-inch x 13-inch casserole dish. Add the soup stock or water. Stir, cover, and bake for about 60 minutes.

All information is per serving:

Calories: 281 (10% from protein, 6% from fat)
Protein: 7.2 gm., Fat: 2.0 gm., Linoleic Acid: .7 gm., Fiber: 2.2 gm.
Calcium: 76 mg., Sodium: 78 mg., Iron: 2.2 mg.
B-Carotene: 6 µg., Vitamin C: 11 mg., Vitamin E: 1.1 mg.
Selenium: .020 mg., Zinc: 2.1 mg.

TOASTED RICE WITH HERBS

preparation time: 20 min.
cooking time: 60 min.

servings: 6

❑ Bring the 5 cups water to a boil in a 4-quart saucepan.

❑ Meanwhile, place the rice and 1 tsp. each of the sage, marjoram, and thyme in a heavy-bottomed sauté pan, and toast over high heat while stirring constantly until the rice is browned evenly.

❑ Add the toasted rice to the boiling water by the spoonful so as not to boil over. Cover and simmer for 35-40 minutes until all the liquid has been absorbed. Remove from the heat, keep covered, and let set for 15 minutes.

❑ Meanwhile, steam-fry the mushrooms and 1 tsp. each of the sage, marjoram, and thyme in 1/4 cup water, juice, or stock for 10 minutes. Add the mushrooms to the cooked rice, and stir to fluff.

5 cups water

3 cups uncooked short grain brown rice
2 tsp. sage
2 tsp. marjoram
2 tsp. thyme

4 cups sliced mushrooms
1/4 cup water, apple-celery juice, or soup stock

All information is per serving:

Calories: 362.7 (9% from protein, 7% from fat)
Protein: 8.2 gm., Fat: 2.8 gm., Linoleic Acid: 1.0 gm., Fiber: 2.2 gm.
Calcium: 55 mg., Sodium: 13 mg., Iron: 3.2 mg.
B-Carotene: n/a, Vitamin C: 2 mg., Vitamin E: .7 mg.
Selenium: .028 mg., Zinc: 2.4 mg.

STUFFED PEPPERS

preparation time: 30 min.
cooking time: 1 hour, 30 min.

servings: 8

5 cups vegetable stock or water
1 1/4 cups uncooked brown rice
1 1/4 cups uncooked millet
2 Tbsp. dried basil
2 tsp. dried oregano
2 cloves garlic, minced

1/2 cup finely chopped celery
1/2 cup diced tomato
1/2 cup mushrooms, sliced

8 red or green bell peppers, tops and
  seeds removed

2 cups Vegetable Marinara Sauce
  (see p. 47)

❑ In a medium pot, bring the water or stock to a boil.

❑ Meanwhile, toast the grains and half the herbs in a nonstick pan over medium-high heat, stirring constantly. Slowly add the toasted grains to the hot stock or water, one spoonful at a time.

❑ Cover and simmer on low heat for 40 minutes. Remove from the heat and keep covered.

❑ Steam-fry the vegetables in 1/2 cup water with the remaining herbs and the garlic for 10 minutes.

❑ Preheat the oven to 350° F. Combine the vegetable mixture with the rice and millet, and spoon into the prepared peppers. Top with the Vegetable Marinara Sauce. Bake for 45 minutes.

All information is per serving:

Calories: 270 (11% from protein, 8% from fat)
Protein: 7.4 gm., Fat: 2.5 gm., Linoleic Acid: 1.1 gm., Fiber: 6.8 gm.
Calcium: 43 mg., Sodium: 25 mg., Iron: 2.6 mg.
B-Carotene: 67 µg., Vitamin C: 65 mg., Vitamin E: .9 mg.
Selenium: .008 mg., Zinc: 1.5 mg.

POTATO PIE

preparation time: 20 min.
cooking time: 60 min.

servings: 4

❑ In a food processor with a shredding blade or with a hand grater, shred the potatoes, then rinse them under cold water in a colander. Combine the potatoes in a mixing bowl with the rice milk or soymilk, flour, and garlic powder.

❑ Preheat the oven to 325° F.

❑ Press half of the potato mixture into a 4-quart baking dish. Layer the vegetables beginning with the greens, then the onions, mushrooms, and bell pepper.

❑ Spread the remaining potatoes over the top. Cover and bake in the preheated oven for 60 minutes. Top with Mushroom Pepper Sauce (see p. 48) or Emerald Sauce (see p. 51).

4 large potatoes, scrubbed
1 cup Rice Milk (see p. 151) or low-fat soymilk
2 Tbsp. oat flour or whole wheat flour
1 tsp. garlic powder

2 cups chopped Swiss chard
2 green onions, sliced
1 1/2 cups sliced mushrooms
1 red or green bell pepper, diced

All information is per serving:

Calories: 309 (11% from protein, 3% from fat)
Protein: 9.2 gm., Fat: 1.0 gm., Linoleic Acid: .3 gm., Fiber: 8.5 gm.
Calcium: 83.6 mg., Sodium: 176 mg., Iron: 5.6 mg.
B-Carotene: 295 µg., Vitamin C: 57.5 mg., Vitamin E: 1.7 mg.
Selenium: .050 mg., Zinc: 1.6 mg.

POLENTA-STUFFED PEPPERS

preparation time: 30 min.
cooking time: 60 min.

servings: 6

3 cups soup stock or water
1/2 cup chopped green onion
2 cups diced mushrooms
8 oz. tomato paste
1 Tbsp. garlic powder
2 Tbsp. basil

1 cup white or yellow cornmeal
6 medium red or green bell peppers

❑ Simmer all the ingredients, except the cornmeal and bell peppers, in a medium pot until the mushrooms are tender.

❑ Cut the tops off the peppers, and remove the centers and seeds. Place snugly, open end up, in a casserole dish.

❑ When the vegetables are done, slowly stir in the cornmeal, and simmer on low heat, stirring constantly, until the polenta starts to thicken (approximately 10 minutes). Spoon the mixture into the peppers until they are full.

❑ Preheat the oven to 350° F. Place 1/2 cup water in the bottom of the casserole dish, cover, and bake for 45-60 minutes. (Check the water periodically and add more if it has steamed away.) Top with Vegetable Marinara Sauce (see p. 47) or gravy, and serve.

All information is per serving:

Calories: 148 (12% from protein, 6% from fat)
Protein: 4.9 gm., Fat: 1.0 gm., Linoleic Acid: .4 gm., Fiber: 3.9 gm.
Calcium: 29 mg., Sodium: 32 mg., Iron: 2.1 mg.
B-Carotene: 64 µg., Vitamin C: 75 mg., Vitamin E: .6 mg.
Selenium: .004 mg., Zinc: .8 mg.

STEAM-FRY VEGETABLES

preparation time: 20 min.
cooking time: 15 min.

servings: 6

❑ Steam-fry all the ingredients, except the bean sprouts and arrowroot, in the stock or juice until just tender (about 15 minutes).

❑ Stir in the bean sprouts for the last 2 minutes of cooking. Remove the vegetables from the liquid, and set aside, keeping warm.

❑ Over medium heat, slowly whisk in the arrowroot, and heat until thick. Pour the sauce over the vegetables, and serve.

6 cups cooked rice
1 red or green bell pepper, diced
2 cups soup stock or celery juice
2 cups apple juice
1 tsp. ginger
1 tsp. garlic powder
3 ribs celery, sliced
1 head broccoli, chopped
1/2 head cauliflower, chopped
2 carrots, sliced
2 cups sliced mushrooms
1 leek or onion, sliced

4 cups mung bean sprouts

1 tsp. arrowroot

All information is per serving:

Calories: 282 (13% from protein, 7% from fat)
Protein: 9.7 gm., Fat: 2.2 gm., Linoleic Acid: .6 gm., Fiber: 10.0 gm.
Calcium: 85 mg., Sodium: 78 mg., Iron: 2.7 mg.
B-Carotene: 688 µg., Vitamin C: 109 mg., Vitamin E: .1 mg.
Selenium: .077 mg., Zinc: 2.1 mg.

BEAN ENTREES

KILLER BLACK BEANS

preparation time: 15 min.
cooking time: 2 hours

servings: 4

---

2 cups dried black beans

4 cups stock, water, or 1 1/2 cups celery juice and 2 1/2 cups water

2 cups chopped mushrooms
4 ribs celery, diced

3 oz. tomato paste
2 cups chopped tomatoes
1 tsp. cumin
1 tsp. oregano
1 Tbsp. garlic powder

❑ Cover the beans with water, and soak overnight. Bring the beans to a boil, adding more water if necessary, then remove from the heat, and drain.

❑ In a 4-quart saucepan, bring the stock, water, or juice and beans to a boil. Lower the heat to medium-low, and simmer until tender (about 70 minutes).

❑ Add the mushrooms and celery, and continue simmering for 20 minutes.

❑ Whisk in the tomato paste, tomatoes, and seasonings. Stir and simmer an additional 20 minutes.

All information is per serving:

Calories: 294 (24% from protein, 5% from fat)
Protein: 18.6 gm., Fat: 1.8 gm., Linoleic Acid: .5 gm., Fiber: 10.2 gm.
Calcium: 119 mg., Sodium: 251 mg., Iron: 31 mg.
B-Carotene: 141 µg., Vitamin C: 31 mg., Vitamin E: .4 mg.
Selenium: .006 mg., Zinc: 2.7 mg.

YAMBURGERS

preparation time: 15 min.
cooking time: 60 min.

servings: 8

❑ In a 4-quart saucepan, bring all the ingredients to a boil, cover, and cook over low heat for 60 minutes, stirring occasionally. Mash and stir to mix the yams thoroughly. Let cool.

❑ Form into 8 patties, and either brown in a nonstick skillet, or place on a nonstick baking sheet, and bake at 375° F until brown.

Hint: Good with Homemade Ketchup (see p. 49).

2 cups water
1 cup dried lentils
1 rib celery, diced
2 large yams, peeled and diced
4 oz. tomato paste
1 tsp. Italian seasoning
1/2 tsp. garlic powder

All information is per serving (1 patty):

Calories: 100 (21% from protein, 3% from fat)

Protein: 5.6 gm., Fat: .4 gm., Linoleic Acid: .1 gm., Fiber: 4.0 gm.

Calcium: 26 mg., Sodium: 19 mg., Iron: 2.2 mg.

B-Carotene: 623 µg., Vitamin C: 14 mg., Vitamin E: 1.4 mg.

Selenium: .005 mg., Zinc: .9 mg.

PINTO BEAN CHILI

preparation time: 10 min.
cooking time: 2 hours, 15 min.

servings: 8

3 cups dried pinto beans
6 cups stock or water
1 cup apple juice

2 leek bulbs, chopped
2 tsp. garlic powder
1 tsp. cumin
1/4 cup fresh cilantro, or 1 Tbsp. dried

24 oz. tomato paste

Optional additions to make chunky:
1 eggplant, chopped
2-4 cups chopped steamed vegetables
3-4 cups chopped fresh tomatoes

❑ Boil the beans in the stock or water and apple juice for 90 minutes.

❑ Add the leeks and spices, and cook until the beans are tender (approximately 30 minutes more).

❑ Add the tomato paste and stir in. Add any optional vegetables and cook for 15 minutes; serve.

All information is per serving:

Calories: 285 (19% from protein, 5% from fat)
Protein: 14.4 gm., Fat: 1.6 gm., Linoleic Acid: .4 gm., Fiber: 13.9 gm.
Calcium: 118 mg., Sodium: 69 mg., Iron: 6.9 mg.
B-Carotene: 3.5 µg., Vitamin C: 43 mg., Vitamin E: .4 mg.
Selenium: .010 mg., Zinc: 2.2 mg.

CRISP VEGGIE MILLET PILAF

preparation time: 45 min.
cooking time: 20 min.

servings: 6

❑ Bring the stock or juice and water to a boil. Meanwhile, sort and rinse the lentils and split peas. Add with the millet to the liquid, return to a boil, then reduce to simmer for 20 minutes. Remove from the heat, cover, and let set for 10-15 minutes.

❑ While the pilaf is cooking, steam-fry the vegetables in 2 Tbsp. of water in the following order—carrots, mushrooms, squash, peas—so that when you are done, each vegetable is tender, yet still crisp and bright. Add the pilaf and mix in.

1 1/2 cups vegetable stock, or the juice from 1 red bell pepper and 8 ribs celery
4 cups water
1/2 cup dried brown or green lentils
1/2 cup dried red lentils
1/4 cup dried green split peas
1/4 cup dried yellow split peas
1 1/2 cups uncooked millet

3 carrots, cut in half lengthwise, thinly sliced (2 cups)
10 button mushrooms, thinly sliced (4 cups)
4 small crookneck squash, sliced 1/4-inch thick (2 cups)
2 cups snap peas, stems and strings removed

All information is per serving:

Calories: 434 (19% from protein, 6% from fat)
Protein: 21.5 gm., Fat: 3.2 gm., Linoleic Acid: 1.4 gm., Fiber: (Gm)19 gm.
Calcium: 99 mg., Sodium: 114 mg., Iron: 7.4 mg.
B-Carotene: 2015 µg., Vitamin C: 29 mg., Vitamin E: 1.1 mg.
Selenium: .018 mg., Zinc: 3.7 mg.

LENTIL LOAF

preparation time: 10 min.
cooking time: 60 min.

servings: 5

---

4 cups Tomato Lentil Stew (see p. 35)
2 cups cooked rice
1/2 cup white or yellow cornmeal
1 cup Vegetable Marinara Sauce (see p. 47)
2 cups steamed vegetables, diced
1 tsp. garlic powder
1 tsp. sage
1 tsp. thyme

❑ Preheat the oven to 350° F. In a large mixing bowl, combine all of the ingredients. Spoon into a loaf pan, cover, and bake for 45-60 minutes.

❑ If served hot, it will spoon out of the pan; if allowed to cool, it can be sliced more like a loaf. Good hot or cold. Serve with Vegetable Marinara Sauce (see p. 47) or any homemade gravy.

All information is per serving:

Calories: 349 (22% from protein, 5% from fat)
Protein: 19.6 gm., Fat: 2.0 gm., Linoleic Acid: .7 gm., Fiber: 13.8 gm.
Calcium: 79 mg., Sodium: 31 mg., Iron: 7.4 mg.
B-Carotene: 106 µg., Vitamin C: 54 mg., Vitamin E: n/a
Selenium: .048 mg., Zinc: 3.1 mg.

YAM LENTIL VEGGIE PATTIES

preparation time: 20 min.
cooking time: 60 min.

servings: 8

❑ Place all the ingredients in an 8-quart pot, and cook over medium heat for 45 minutes until the lentils and rice are soft. Let cool.

❑ Form into 8 patties. Brown in a nonstick frying pan, or broil on a nonstick baking sheet until browned.

5 cups water
1 cup dried lentils
2 cups diced yams
1/4 cup uncooked short grain brown rice
1/4 cup uncooked wild rice
1/2 cup white or yellow cornmeal
1/2 cup minced celery
1/2 cup shredded carrots
1/2 cup diced zucchini

All information is per serving (1 patty):

Calories: 168 (16% from protein, 4% from fat)
Protein: 7.0 gm., Fat: .7 gm., Linoleic Acid: .3 gm., Fiber: 4.8 gm.
Calcium: 54 mg., Sodium: 113 mg., Iron: 2.6 mg.
B-Carotene: 757 µg., Vitamin C: 6.5 mg., Vitamin E: 1.7 mg.
Selenium: .007 mg., Zinc: 1.3 mg.

MIDDLE EASTERN GOULASH

preparation time: 20 min.
cooking time: 60 min.

servings: 10

8 1/2 cups water or soup stock
2 cups dried lentils
2 cups uncooked rice
1/2 cup uncooked wild rice
1 yam, peeled and diced
1 Tbsp. garlic powder
1 Tbsp. cumin
1 Tbsp. parsley flakes
juice of 1 lemon

3 carrots, julienned or grated
3 ribs celery, julienned or grated

❑ Bring the water or soup stock to a boil in a 4-quart saucepan. Add the lentils, rice, yam, spices, and lemon juice.

❑ Return to a boil, then simmer on medium-low for 25 minutes. Add the carrots and celery, and simmer for 20 more minutes.

❑ Remove from the heat, cover, and let set for 15 minutes. Mix gently and serve.

Hint: This recipe can be cooked by adding all the ingredients at one time for easier preparation.

All information is per serving:

Calories: 308 (16% from protein, 5% from fat)
Protein: 12.3 gm., Fat: 1.7 gm., Linoleic Acid: .5 gm., Fiber: 6.1 gm.
Calcium: 57 mg., Sodium: 32 mg., Iron: 4.3 mg.
B-Carotene: 1056 µg., Vitamin C: 11 mg., Vitamin E: 1.8 mg.
Selenium: .018 mg., Zinc: 2.5 mg.

DILLED CARROT CUTLETS

preparation time: 15 min.
cooking time: 20 min.

servings: 7

❑ Preheat the oven to 350° F. Blend all the ingredients in a food processor until smooth, and shape into 7 small patties.

❑ Bake on a nonstick baking sheet for 10 minutes on each side.

2 cups cooked white beans
1 1/2 carrots, grated
1/3 cup cooked rice or millet
1/3 cup celery juice or water
1 Tbsp. dill weed

All information is per serving (1 patty):

Calories: 94 (23% from protein, 3% from fat)

Protein: 5.7 gm., Fat: .4 gm., Linoleic Acid: .1 gm., Fiber: 3.7 gm.

Calcium: 60 mg., Sodium: 24 mg., Iron: 2.2 mg.

B-Carotene: 436 μg., Vitamin C: 3 mg., Vitamin E: .3 mg.

Selenium: n/a, Zinc: .9 mg.

EASY SPLIT PEA LOAF

preparation time: 10 min.
cooking time: 60 min.

servings: 6

6 cups Split Pea and Yam Soup
   (see p. 24)
approximately 1 cup soup stock, celery
   juice, or water
1 cup white or yellow cornmeal

❑ Preheat the oven to 350° F. In a food processor, blend the soup with enough of the stock, juice, or water to thin to a "tomato soup" consistency. Place in a bowl and stir in the cornmeal.

❑ Pour the mixture into a loaf pan, and bake for 60 minutes, or until a toothpick inserted in the center comes out clean.

❑ Allow to cool for slicing, or serve by the spoonful like a stuffing.

Variation: Use any leftover bean or pea soup.

All information is per serving:

Calories: 225 (17% from protein, 3% from fat)

Protein: 9.6 gm., Fat: .8 gm., Linoleic Acid: .3 gm., Fiber: 3.6 gm.

Calcium: 35 mg., Sodium: 20 mg., Iron: 1.8 mg.

B-Carotene: 511 µg., Vitamin C: 11 mg., Vitamin E: 1.3 mg.

Selenium: .002 mg., Zinc: 1.2 mg.

LIMA BEANS

preparation time: 15 min.
cooking time: 45 min.

servings: 6

❑ Soak the beans overnight, boil, and drain. Cook about 2 hours in the stock or water.

❑ In a 4-quart saucepan, bring all the ingredients, except the herbs, to a boil.

❑ Reduce to medium heat and simmer for 35 minutes. Add the herbs and simmer for 10 more minutes.

2 cups dried lima beans
8 cups stock or water

1 cup diced celery
2 large yams, peeled and diced

1 tsp. thyme
1 tsp. savory
1/4 cup chopped fresh parsley

All information is per serving:

Calories: 183 (23% from protein, 3% from fat)
Protein: 10.8 gm., Fat: .7 gm., Linoleic Acid: .034 gm., Fiber: 7.9 gm.
Calcium: 119 mg., Sodium: 35 mg., Iron: 3.3 mg.
B-Carotene: 832 µg., Vitamin C: 16 mg., Vitamin E: 2.1 mg.
Selenium: .016 mg., Zinc: 1.3 mg.

ORIENTAL LENTILS

preparation time: 15 min.
cooking time: 35 min.

servings: 5

4 cups water
2 cups dried lentils
1-2 tsp. ground ginger
1 Tbsp. garlic powder

1 1/2 cups mung bean sprouts
1 1/2 cups sliced mushrooms
1 1/2 cups sliced celery

❑ In a 2-quart saucepan, bring the water to a boil. Add the lentils, ginger, and garlic, then simmer for 25 minutes. Add more water if necessary to keep from sticking.

❑ Pour the cooked lentils into a sauté pan with the vegetables, and simmer for 10 minutes.

All information is per serving:

Calories: 206 (30% from protein, 3% from fat)
Protein: 16 gm., Fat: .8 gm., Linoleic Acid: .3 gm., Fiber: 8.6 gm.
Calcium: 38 mg., Sodium: 9.3 mg., Iron: 5.9 mg.
B-Carotene: 2.2 µg., Vitamin C: 7.2 mg., Vitamin E: .2 mg.
Selenium: .019 mg., Zinc: 2.4 mg.

BLACK-EYED PEAS

preparation time: 15 min.
cooking time: 1 hour, 30 min.

servings: 5

❑ In a 4-quart saucepan, bring all the ingredients to a boil. Cover and cook over low heat for 90 minutes, or until the peas are tender. Stir occasionally.

Variation: Try green or yellow split peas instead of the black-eyed peas.

2 cups dried black-eyed peas
8 1/2 cups water or stock
1 cup diced yam or sweet potato
1 medium russet potato, diced
1 cup diced celery
1 cup diced carrots
1/2 cup fresh parsley, minced, or 2 Tbsp. dried
1/2 tsp. celery seed
1/2 tsp. thyme
1/4 tsp. marjoram

All information is per serving:

Calories: 146 (11% from protein, 3% from fat)

Protein: 4.1 gm., Fat: .5 gm., Linoleic Acid: .2 gm., Fiber: 8.0 gm.

Calcium: 136 mg., Sodium: 76 mg., Iron: 2.0 mg.

B-Carotene: 1217 µg., Vitamin C: 16 mg., Vitamin E: 1.8 mg.

Selenium: n/a, Zinc: 1.2 mg.

123

FALAFEL

preparation time: 15 min.
cooking time: 30 min.

servings: 6

4 cups cooked garbanzo beans
2 cups cooked brown rice
2 ribs celery, diced
1/2 red or green bell pepper, chopped
2 tomatoes, chopped
juice of 1 lemon
1 Tbsp. basil
1 Tbsp. garlic powder
2 tsp. cumin

❑ Purée all the ingredients until smooth in a food processor.

❑ Drop by spoonfuls onto a nonstick frying pan, and cook over medium heat until brown (about 15 minutes). Flip over and brown the other side. Serve hot or cold.

All information is per serving:
Calories: 335 (19% from protein, 11% from fat)
Protein: 16.4 gm., Fat: 4.2 gm., Linoleic Acid: .3 gm., Fiber: 2.0 gm.
Calcium: 125 mg., Sodium: 38 mg., Iron: 5.7 mg.
B-Carotene: 1.7 µg., Vitamin C: 15 mg., Vitamin E: .5 mg.
Selenium: .027 mg., Zinc: .6 mg.

GARBANZO BEAN LOAF

preparation time: 15 min.
cooking time: 30 min.

servings: 8

❑ Preheat the oven to 350° F. In a large mixing bowl, combine the blended beans and rice. Add the tomato sauce, mustard, carrots, and lemon juice.

❑ Spoon into a loaf pan, and bake for 30 minutes. Cover the loaf with aluminum foil if the top begins to brown too quickly.

Variation: Add 1 1/2 tsp. garlic powder or onion powder with the other seasonings.

4 cups cooked, blended garbanzo beans
2 cups cooked brown rice
2 cups tomato sauce
1 Tbsp. dry mustard
1 cup grated carrots
juice of 1/2 lemon

All information is per serving:

Calories: 264 (18% from protein, 10% from fat)
Protein: 12.3 gm., Fat: 3.1 gm., Linoleic Acid: .2 gm., Fiber: 2.2 gm.
Calcium: 98 mg., Sodium: 31 mg., Iron: 4.4 mg.
B-Carotene: 98 μg., Vitamin C: 11 mg., Vitamin E: .2 mg.
Selenium: .022 mg., Zinc: .5 mg.

EXCELLENT POLENTA BEAN PIE

preparation time: 45 min.
cooking time: 2 hours

servings: 8

Crust:
12 oz. tomato paste
5 1/2 cups water or vegetable stock
1 rib celery, diced
1 red bell pepper, chopped
2 tsp. cumin
1 Tbsp. garlic powder
3 Tbsp. minced fresh cilantro

2 cups white or yellow cornmeal

Filling:
4 cups water
2 cups dried black beans
3 ribs celery, diced

1 red or green bell pepper, diced
kernels from 2 ears fresh corn
1/2 onion, minced
1 tsp. cumin
2 tsp. oregano
1 Tbsp. garlic powder
2 Tbsp. minced fresh cilantro
8 oz. tomato paste

❑ To make the crust, simmer the tomato paste, 2 cups of the water or stock, the 1 rib of celery, chopped red bell pepper, cumin, 1 Tbsp. garlic powder, and 3 Tbsp. cilantro in a 4-quart saucepan.

❑ To make the polenta, bring the remaining water to a boil in another 4-quart saucepan. Slowly sprinkle the cornmeal into the boiling water, stirring continuously until it starts to pull away from the sides of the pan.

❑ Preheat the oven to 350° F. Add the tomato sauce mixture, and stir well. Transfer this polenta mixture into a 4-quart baking dish. Cover with foil and bake for 60 minutes, or until firm. Let cool.

❑ To make the filling, simmer the 4 cups water, beans, and 3 ribs celery for 60 minutes in an 8-quart soup pot over medium-high heat.

❑ Add the remaining vegetables and spices, and cook for 30 more minutes.

❑ Add the tomato paste and cook for 30 minutes. Remove half of the beans, and purée in a blender or food processor. Pour the remaining whole beans over the cooled polenta crust.

❑ Top with the puréed beans, and decorate as desired with sliced tomato, fresh cilantro leaves, etc. Bake at 375° F for 15 minutes. Let cool and serve.

Hint: The puréed beans also make a superb dip for baked tortilla chips.

All information is per serving:

Calories: 218 (16% from protein, 7% from fat)

Protein: 9.6 gm., Fat: 1.8 gm., Linoleic Acid: .7 gm., Fiber: 8.4 gm.

Calcium: 55 mg., Sodium: 56 mg., Iron: 4 mg.

B-Carotene: 7.8 µg., Vitamin C: 31 mg., Vitamin E: .2 mg.

Selenium: .001 mg., Zinc: 1.6 mg.

CAJUN BLACK BEAN GUMBO

preparation time: 35 min.
cooking time: approximately 2 hours

servings: 12

4 cups dried black beans

10 cups soup stock
4 bay leaves

1 bunch green onions, minced
2 carrots, diced
6 ribs celery, diced
2 red or green bell peppers, diced
1 tsp. oregano
1 tsp. thyme

10 button mushrooms, sliced
6 cups diced fresh tomatoes
15 small okra, sliced into rounds
kernels from 3 ears fresh corn

❑ Soak the beans overnight in enough water to cover. Boil for 5 minutes and drain.

❑ In an 8-quart soup pot, add the soup stock and bay leaves, and simmer the beans over medium heat for 90 minutes.

❑ Meanwhile, steam-fry the onions in 1 cup water for 3-5 minutes. Stir in the carrots, celery, bell peppers, oregano, and thyme, then cook for another 10 minutes, adding liquid as needed.

❑ Add the mushrooms and tomatoes, and simmer 5 more minutes, then remove from heat.

❑ Once the beans are cooked, add the vegetable mixture and stir well. Finally, add the okra and corn kernels, and simmer until tender (about 10 minutes).

All information is per serving:

Calories: 205 (23% from protein, 5% from fat)
Protein: 12.3 gm., Fat: 1.2 gm., Linoleic Acid: .3 gm., Fiber: 7.5 gm.
Calcium: 481 mg., Sodium: 40 mg., Iron: 3.6 mg.
B-Carotene: 481 µg., Vitamin C: 38 mg., Vitamin E: 7 mg.
Selenium: .002 mg., Zinc: 1.7 mg.

SIDE DISHES

BLACK JAPONICA PILAF

preparation time: 20 min.
cooking time: 40 min.

servings: 5

2 cups vegetable stock or celery-red
   pepper juice (made from 1 red bell
   pepper and 7 ribs celery)
2 cups water
1 cup uncooked millet
1/2 cup uncooked short grain brown
   rice
1/2 cup uncooked black japonica rice
1 tsp. garlic powder
1/2 tsp. oregano
1/2 tsp. cumin

❑ Bring the stock or juice and water to a boil in a medium saucepan. Add the grains and seasonings, stir, return to a boil, cover, and simmer for 35 minutes.

❑ Remove from the heat and let set covered for another 15 minutes. Remove the lid, fluff evenly with a fork, and serve.

Variation: Add 1/2 cup raisins and/or chopped walnuts after cooking.

All information is per serving:

Calories: 305 (10% from protein, 9% from fat)
Protein: 8.0 gm., Fat: 2.9 gm., Linoleic Acid: 1.2 gm., Fiber: 7.6 gm.
Calcium: 47 mg., Sodium: 56 mg., Iron: 2.4 mg.
B-Carotene: 15 µg., Vitamin C: 17 mg., Vitamin E: .6 mg.
Selenium: .009 mg., Zinc: 1.6 mg.

EGGPLANT PÂTÉ

preparation time: 20 min.
cooking time: 30 min.

servings: 6

❑ Preheat the oven to 350° F. Pierce the eggplant with fork in eight places to allow steam to escape. Place on a baking sheet, and bake for 30 minutes. Allow to cool completely.

❑ When the eggplant is cool, remove the skin, and combine the pulp, tahini, lemon juice, parsley, and garlic. Blend in a food processor until smooth. Pâté can be used as a dip or a spread.

1 medium eggplant

3/4 cup raw sesame tahini
juice of 1/2 lemon
1/2 cup chopped fresh parsley
1 clove garlic, minced, or 1/4 tsp. garlic powder (optional)

All information is per serving:

Calories: 124 (12% from protein, 61% from fat)
Protein: 3.9 gm., Fat: 9.1 gm., Linoleic Acid: 3.9 gm., Fiber: 4.6 gm.
Calcium: 187 mg., Sodium: 7 mg., Iron: 3.2 mg.
B-Carotene: 6 μg., Vitamin C: 10 mg., Vitamin E: .5 mg.
Selenium: n/a, Zinc: 1.5 mg.

DAL

preparation time: 30 min.
cooking time: 60 min.

servings: 9

6 cups water
3 cups dried split peas or red lentils

2 carrots, diced
2 ribs celery, diced
juice of 1 lemon
2 tsp. cumin
1 Tbsp. garlic granules
1 tsp. onion powder
1/2 tsp. dry mustard
1/2 tsp. turmeric
1/4 tsp. cloves

1 tsp. minced fresh cilantro, or 1/2 tsp.
  dry

❑ In a 4-quart saucepan, bring the water to a boil. Add the split peas or lentils, and simmer for 45 minutes, stirring occasionally.

❑ In a 10-inch skillet, steam-fry the carrots, celery, lemon juice, and seasonings, except for the fresh cilantro, until tender, adding water as needed to keep the vegetables from sticking to the pan.

❑ Stir the steamed vegetables into the split peas or lentils, and cook an additional 15 minutes. Sprinkle with fresh cilantro.

Hint: If using dry cilantro, add to the vegetables with the other seasonings.

All information is per serving:

Calories: 236 (27% from protein, 4% from fat)
Protein: 16.6 gm., Fat: 1.0 gm., Linoleic Acid: .3 gm., Fiber: 2.9 gm.
Calcium: 53 mg., Sodium: 24 mg., Iron: 5.4 mg.
B-Carotene: 2.4 µg., Vitamin C: 5 mg., Vitamin E: .3 mg.
Selenium: .001 mg., Zinc: 2.1 mg.

APPLE-RAISIN CHUTNEY

preparation time: 15 min.
cooking time: 40 min.

servings: 6

❑ Combine all the ingredients in a 2-quart saucepan. Cook uncovered on low for 40 minutes. Serve warm or chilled.

3 apples, peeled, cored, and diced
1/2 cup raisins
1 cup minced celery
1 Tbsp. tarragon
1/4 cup apple cider vinegar
1 Tbsp. lemon juice
1 tsp. ginger

All information is per serving:

Calories: 82 (4% from protein, 4% from fat)

Protein: .9 gm., Fat: .4 gm., Linoleic Acid: .1 gm., Fiber: 1.8 gm.

Calcium: 27 mg., Sodium: 20 mg., Iron: .7 mg.

B-Carotene: 5.8 µg., Vitamin C: 5.5 mg., Vitamin E: .3 mg.

Selenium: .001 mg., Zinc: .1 mg.

CORN BREAD

preparation time: 10 min.
cooking time: 30 min.

servings: 12

1 1/2 cups apple juice
2 cups cornmeal
1 cup oat flour (can be oatmeal ground
  in a blender or food processor)
4 tsp. baking powder
1/2 cup applesauce

❑ Preheat the oven to 325° F. Warm the apple juice in a 2-quart saucepan just until hot, but not boiling. Mix all the dry ingredients together, then add the applesauce and warm apple juice.

❑ Stir just until moistened, and pour into an 8-inch x 10-inch nonstick baking pan. Bake for 30 minutes.

Hint: This is a hearty bread best served with a favorite soup.

All information is per serving:

Calories: 140 (11% from protein, 10% from fat)
Protein: 3.9 gm., Fat: 1.7 gm., Linoleic Acid: .6 gm., Fiber: 5.1 gm.
Calcium: 82 mg., Sodium: 10 mg., Iron: 1.5 mg.
B-Carotene: .3 µg., Vitamin C: 1 mg., Vitamin E: .2 mg.
Selenium: .004 mg., Zinc: .9 mg.

BRAISED RED CABBAGE

preparation time: 15 min.
cooking time: 45-60 min.

servings: 4

❑ Place all the ingredients in a 4-quart saucepan, and steam-fry over high heat for 5 minutes, stirring occasionally.

❑ Lower the heat to medium-low, and simmer uncovered for 45 minutes, or until the cabbage is soft, stirring occasionally.

❑ Add water or more apple juice as needed to keep the vegetables from sticking to the pan.

8 cups shredded red cabbage (1 small head)
1 small onion, or 2 tsp. onion powder
2 tart apples, peeled, cored, and diced
2 cups apple juice
1/4 tsp. ground cloves
2 tsp. apple cider vinegar
1 bay leaf

All information is per serving:

Calories: 121 (4% from protein, 4% from fat)
Protein: 1.4 gm., Fat: .6 gm., Linoleic Acid: .1 gm., Fiber: 3.6 gm.
Calcium: 54 mg., Sodium: 13 mg., Iron: 1.0 mg.
B-Carotene: 8 μg., Vitamin C: 41 mg., Vitamin E: 2.0 mg.
Selenium: .008 mg., Zinc: .2 mg.

BAKED TOMATOES

preparation time: 10 min.
cooking time: 20 min.

servings: 4

4 medium tomatoes, halved widthwise
2 Tbsp. parsley flakes
2 Tbsp. minced chives or scallions
1 Tbsp. basil
1/2 cup apple juice

❑ Preheat the oven to 325° F. Place the halved tomatoes, cut side up, in a shallow, nonstick baking pan. Sprinkle the parsley, chives, basil, and apple juice over the tomatoes.

❑ Bake until tender (about 20 minutes).

All information is per serving:

Calories: 45 (11% from protein, 9% from fat)

Protein: 1.4 gm., Fat: .5 gm., Linoleic Acid: .2 gm., Fiber: 1.7 gm.

Calcium: 38 mg., Sodium: 14 mg., Iron: 1.6 mg.

B-Carotene: 141 µg., Vitamin C: 26 mg., Vitamin E: .4 mg.

Selenium: .001 mg., Zinc: .2 mg.

VEGETABLE SOUP STOCK

preparation time: 10 min.
cooking time: 30 min.

❑ Use enough water to cover the amount of vegetables you use.

❑ Using a large, covered pot, cook over medium heat about 30 minutes. Strain the stock immediately, cool, and refrigerate.

❑ The stock can be frozen in single serving containers.

Hints: If you need stock in a hurry, try juicing leftover steamed vegetables or using the water leftover in a pot after steaming vegetables.

Depending on the freezer space available, you can make as much stock as you like.

Avoid cabbage, broccoli, cauliflower, and brussel sprouts; these vegetables can overpower the flavor of the stock.

Basic ingredients:
carrots
celery
onion
garlic
tomatoes
bay leaves

POTATO SALAD

preparation time: 20 min.
cooking time: 15 min.

servings: 8

12 cups red creamer potatoes, cut into
  1-inch cubes
1 cup celery juice or vegetable stock
3 cups water

3 ribs celery, diced
2 carrots, diced
1 red or green bell pepper, diced
1/2 cup diced green onions
1 1/2 Tbsp. dill weed
1 tsp. basil
1/2 tsp. garlic powder
1/2 tsp. onion powder

❑ In a 4-quart saucepan, simmer the potatoes in the juice or stock and water until just tender. Allow to cool.

❑ In a large mixing bowl, combine the remaining ingredients, and let stand to marry the flavors.

❑ When the potatoes are cool, mix all the ingredients together, and serve.

All information is per serving:

Calories: 317 (8% from protein, 1% from fat)
Protein: 6.6 gm., Fat: .5 gm., Linoleic Acid: .1 gm., Fiber: 5.5 gm.
Calcium: 55 mg., Sodium: 44 mg., Iron: 1.6 mg.
B-Carotene: 526 µg., Vitamin C: 37 mg., Vitamin E: .4 mg.
Selenium: .001 mg., Zinc: 1.1 mg.

WILD MUSHROOM SAUTÉ

preparation time: 15 min.
cooking time: 10 min.

servings: 6

❑ In a sauté pan, steam-fry the mush-rooms and peppers in 2 Tbsp. of water for 5 minutes. (This will be enough water as the mushrooms will release a lot of their own liquid.)

❑ Add the spinach and continue stirring for 5 more minutes until the spinach is bright green and just tender.

8 cups sliced crimini mushrooms or any other edible mushrooms
2 red or green bell peppers, diced

1 bunch spinach, well washed, stems removed, and chopped

All information is per serving:

Calories: 34 (26% from protein, 11% from fat)
Protein: 2.7 gm., Fat: .5 gm., Linoleic Acid: .2 gm., Fiber: 2.1 gm.
Calcium: 25 mg., Sodium: 19 mg., Iron: 1.8 mg.
B-Carotene: 138 µg., Vitamin C: 31 mg., Vitamin E: .6 mg.
Selenium: .012 mg., Zinc: .8 mg.

139

TOFU-SPINACH DIP

preparation time: 15 min.
chilling time: 2-4 hours

servings: 6 (makes 2 cups)

2 cups spinach, well washed, stems
  removed, chopped
1 (10.5 oz.) pkg. firm silken tofu,
  drained
1 1/2 Tbsp. lemon juice
3 Tbsp. chopped green onion
1/2 tsp. garlic powder
1/4 tsp. cumin
2 Tbsp. fresh savory

❑ Steam the spinach 2-3 minutes.

❑ In a food processor, purée all the ingredients until smooth. Chill for 2-4 hours.

❑ Serve as dip with fresh vegetables or as
a sandwich spread.

All information is per serving: (1/3 cup)

Calories: 152 (37% from protein, 29% from fat)
Protein: 5.4 gm., Fat: 1.9 gm., Linoleic Acid: .010 gm., Fiber: 11.4 gm.
Calcium: 178 mg., Sodium: 256 mg., Iron: 3.8 mg.
B-Carotene: 1416 µg., Vitamin C: 210 mg., Vitamin E: 1.1 mg.
Selenium: .001 mg., Zinc: 1.5 mg.

SALSA

preparation time: 30 min.
chilling time: 2 hours

servings: 8 (makes about 5 cups)

- ❑ Thoroughly mix all the ingredients together in a large bowl. Cover and refrigerate for at least 2 hours.
- ❑ Serve with raw vegetables, corn tortillas, as a salad dressing, or on veggie burgers.

6 medium-ripe tomatoes, diced
1 red onion, minced
2 dry ancho chiles, seeds removed and minced
1 mild green chile, minced
1 clove garlic, minced, or 1/2 tsp. powder
1 bunch cilantro, finely chopped (1 to 1 1/2 cups)
1/2 cup apple cider vinegar
1 Tbsp. cumin
1 tsp. oregano

All information is per serving (2/3 cup):

Calories: 29 (13% from protein, 13% from fat)
Protein: 1.1 gm., Fat: .5 gm., Linoleic Acid: .1 gm., Fiber: 1.3 gm.
Calcium: 20 mg., Sodium: 11 mg., Iron: 1.2 mg.
B-Carotene: 104 µg., Vitamin C: 19 mg., Vitamin E: .3 mg.
Selenium: .001 mg., Zinc: .1 mg.

NO-FAT FRIES

preparation time: 15 min.
cooking time: 20-30 min.

servings: 4

6 russet potatoes (for variety, try purple potatoes)

❑ Preheat the oven to 425° F. Peel or scrub the potatoes well. Cut into 1/4-inch fries. Use a nonstick baking sheet, or dampen the sheet with water and coat with corn flour.

❑ Spread the fries evenly, and bake for 20 minutes. Test to see if tender. Serve with Homemade Ketchup (see p. 49).

All information is per serving:

Calories: 330 (8% from protein, 1% from fat)
Protein: 7.0 gm., Fat: .3 gm., Linoleic Acid: 1 gm., Fiber: 7.6 gm.
Calcium: 30 mg., Sodium: 24 mg., Iron: 4.1 mg.
B-Carotene: n/a, Vitamin C: 39 mg., Vitamin E: 1 mg.
Selenium: .002 mg., Zinc: 1.0 mg.

HUMMUS-STUFFED CHARD LEAVES

preparation time: 45 min.
chilling time: 60 min.

servings: 10

❑ Place the rice, basil, celery, bell pepper, tomatoes, and lemon juice in a bowl, and mix together.

❑ Spread out the lightly steamed chard leaves one at a time, and place a teaspoonful each of the rice mix and hummus and a few pieces of avocado on the end of the leaf.

❑ Roll up like a burrito, tucking the sides in before rolling completely. Chill and serve.

1 cup cooked brown rice
1 Tbsp. basil
1/4 cup diced celery
1/4 cup diced red or green bell pepper
2 tomatoes, diced
2 Tbsp. lemon juice

1 cup Healthy Hummus (see p. 144)
**10 large chard or kale leaves, steamed
  lightly**
1/2 avocado, diced

All information is per serving:

Calories: 83 (14% from protein, 23% from fat)

Protein: 3.2 gm., Fat: 2.2 gm., Linoleic Acid: .3 gm., Fiber: 1.6 gm.

Calcium: 34 mg., Sodium: 44 mg., Iron: 1.4 mg.

B-Carotene: 80 µg., Vitamin C: 17 mg., Vitamin E: .7 mg.

Selenium: .008 mg., Zinc: .3 mg.

HEALTHY HUMMUS

preparation time: 20 min.

servings: 6

---

4 cups cooked garbanzo beans, well drained
1 1/4 cups vegetable stock or celery juice, and extra as needed for a creamy texture
juice of 1 1/2 lemons
1/2 tsp. garlic powder
1/2 tsp. ground cumin

10 large, fresh basil leaves, finely chopped, or 2 Tbsp. dried
1/2 Tbsp. parsley flakes, or handful of fresh cut leaves (optional)

❑ Blend the beans, stock or celery juice, lemon juice, garlic, and cumin in a food processor until smooth.

❑ Transfer into a bowl, and mix in the minced basil and parsley. Chill and serve.

❑ Garnish with additional basil leaves and/or diced tomatoes.

All information is per serving:

Calories: 195 (21% from protein, 11% from fat)
Protein: 11 gm., Fat: 2.5 gm., Linoleic Acid: .1 gm., Fiber: 1.1 gm.
Calcium: 106 mg., Sodium: 66 mg., Iron: 3.8 mg.
B-Carotene: 7.8 µg., Vitamin C: 12 mg., Vitamin E: .2 mg.
Selenium: .001 mg., Zinc: .1 mg.

SPRING ROLLS

preparation time: 45 min.
cooking time: 10 min.

servings: 8

2 cups mung bean sprouts
1 clove garlic, minced, or 1/2 tsp. powder
1/2 cup apple juice
1 cup celery juice or vegetable stock
1 cup cooked wild rice or long grain brown rice

8 large Swiss chard or kale leaves, cleaned

❑ Steam-fry the bean sprouts and garlic in the apple juice and 1/2 cup of the celery juice or stock for 10 minutes. Drain the steaming liquid and set aside. Gently mix the rice in with the sprouts.

❑ Steam the chard or kale leaves until just wilted (about 5 minutes). Lay them flat and cut the stem to the base of the leaf.

❑ Assemble by placing 1 Tbsp. of the sprout mixture at the tip of the leaf and tightly rolling to the base, creating a tube.

❑ Preheat the oven to 350° F. Place the rolls seam-side-down next to each other in a shallow baking dish. Cover with the remaining sauté liquid and the remaining 1/2 cup of celery juice or stock.

❑ Bake for 10 minutes; do not overcook. Serve as an appetizer or main dish.

All information is per serving (1 roll):

Calories: 61 (18% from protein, 3% from fat)
Protein: 3.0 gm., Fat: .2 gm., Linoleic Acid: .1 gm., Fiber: 1.6 gm.
Calcium: 34 mg., Sodium: 72 mg., Iron: 1.1 mg.
B-Carotene: 73 µg., Vitamin C: 10 mg., Vitamin E: .5 mg.
Selenium: .009 mg., Zinc: .8 mg.

ROASTED RED BELL PEPPERS

preparation time: 15 min.
cooking time: 30 min.
chilling time: 30 min.

red bell peppers

❑ Preheat the oven to broil. Place the peppers 4-6 inches from the heat. Turn to roast all sides of the peppers.

❑ Broil until the peppers are charred (this will take about 30 minutes). Remove the peppers from the oven, and place them in a paper bag.

❑ Refrigerate the roasted peppers until they are cool enough to handle. Remove them from the bag, peel, and remove the seeds.

❑ Use roasted red peppers in casseroles, soups, salads, and sandwiches, or use as a garnish.

ORIENTAL RICE SALAD

preparation time: 20 min.

servings: 3

4 cups cooked short grain brown rice, cooled to room temperature
1 cup finely shredded carrots
1/2 cup raw sunflower seeds
juice of 1/2 lemon
1/2 tsp. ground ginger
1/2 tsp. garlic powder
1/4 cup dulse (seaweed), rinsed

1 red or green bell pepper, diced
1 cucumber, peeled and diced

❑ Toss the ingredients together, except for the bell pepper and cucumber.

❑ Toss the bell pepper and cucumber into the rice mixture. Serve cold or at room temperature.

Hint: You can also use this mixture as a filling for sushi by cutting the pepper and cucumber into thin strips and using them as center vegetables for the sushi roll.

All information is per serving:

Calories: 486 (11% from protein, 26% from fat)
Protein: 13.7 gm., Fat: 14.5 gm., Linoleic Acid: 8.7 gm., Fiber: 8.3 gm.
Calcium: 98 mg., Sodium: 38 mg., Iron: 4.1 mg.
B-Carotene: 2001 µg., Vitamin C: 39 mg., Vitamin E: 14.53 mg.
Selenium: .1 mg., Zinc: 3.3 mg.

MILLET BALLS

preparation time: 10 min.
cooking time: 30 min.

servings: 10

2 cups mashed cooked yams or
   potatoes
4 cups cooked millet (1 1/2 cups millet
   cooked in 4 cups carrot-celery juice
   or soup stock)
1/2 tsp. ground thyme

❑ Preheat the oven to 350° F. Mix all the ingredients in a large mixing bowl with a hand masher. Shape into ten 2-inch balls.

❑ Place on a nonstick baking sheet, and bake for 30 minutes.

All information is per serving (1 ball):

Calories: 178 (11% from protein, 6% from fat)
Protein: 4.8 gm., Fat: 1.1 gm., Linoleic Acid: .5 gm., Fiber: 8.0 gm.
Calcium: 30 mg., Sodium: 34 mg., Iron: 1.3 mg.
B-Carotene: 2533 µg., Vitamin C: 8 mg., Vitamin E: 1.5 mg.
Selenium: n/a, Zinc: 1.1 mg.

Stuffed Mushrooms

preparation time: 45 min.
cooking time: 10-40 min.

servings: 18

❑ Remove the stems of the button mushrooms and chop. Save the whole caps for stuffing. Steam-fry the mushroom stems, shiitake, chard, and leeks in the celery juice or stock and apple juice for 10 minutes. Drain off the juice and save.

❑ Add the basil, garlic, and bread crumbs or cornmeal to the mushrooms. Mix well and stuff the mushroom caps full with this mixture.

❑ Preheat the oven to 350° F. Pour the reserved juices into a shallow pan. Place the stuffed caps face up in the pan, and cover.

❑ Bake for 10-15 minutes if using bread crumbs, 30-40 minutes if using cornmeal. Uncover when done and brown for a few minutes under the broiler.

18 large button mushrooms
1 1/2 cups shiitake mushrooms, chopped
1 cup fresh chard or spinach, chopped
1/2 cup leeks, chopped
1 1/2 cups celery juice or vegetable stock
1 1/2 cups apple juice

1 Tbsp. fresh basil leaves, minced
1/2 Tbsp. garlic powder
1/2 cup whole grain bread crumbs, or
　1/2 cup white or yellow cornmeal

All information is per serving (1 mushroom):

Calories: 42 (11% from protein, 6% from fat)
Protein: 1.2 gm., Fat: .3 gm., Linoleic Acid: .1 gm., Fiber: 1.9 gm.
Calcium: 20 mg., Sodium: 40 mg., Iron: .9 mg.
B-Carotene: 34 µg., Vitamin C: 4.3 mg., Vitamin E: .4 mg.
Selenium: .005 mg., Zinc: .4 mg.

THREE GRAIN STUFFING

preparation time: 25 min.
cooking time: 60 min.

servings: 8

1 3/4 cups uncooked brown rice
1 cup white or yellow cornmeal
1/4 cup uncooked wild rice
4 cups sliced mushrooms
2 1/2 cups diced celery
1/2 cup chopped chives (optional)
1 cup Rice Milk (see p. 151), or low-fat
  soymilk
1 cup apple juice
4 cups soup stock or water

Optional ingredients:
  1 medium apple, cored and chopped
  1 medium yam, peeled and chopped
  1/2 cup raisins
  4 Tbsp. onion powder, or 1 onion,
    diced
  1 Tbsp. sage
  1 Tbsp. thyme

❑ Preheat the oven to 350° F. In a large mixing bowl, combine all of the ingredients, adding the liquids last. Stir well.

❑ Spoon into a covered 4-quart casserole dish. Bake for 60 minutes.

All information is per serving:

Calories: 266 (10% from protein, 7% from fat)
Protein: 6.6 gm., Fat: 2.2 gm., Linoleic Acid: .8 gm., Fiber: 6.0 gm.
Calcium: 37 mg., Sodium: 47 mg., Iron: 2 mg.
B-Carotene: 4.9 µg., Vitamin C: 6 mg., Vitamin E: .6 mg.
Selenium: .019 mg., Zinc: 1.8 mg.

RICE MILK

preparation time: 5 min.

servings: 2 (makes 2 cups)

❑ Purée the rice and water in a blender or food processor, and strain through a very fine strainer, several times if necessary, to remove any grittiness.

Hint: For desserts and when using with cereals, try adding 1/2 tsp. of vanilla.

1 cup cooked brown rice
2 cups water

All information is per serving (1 cup):

Calories: 109 (8% from protein, 7% from fat)

Protein: 2.3 gm., Fat: .8 gm., Linoleic Acid: .3 gm., Fiber: 1.7 gm.

Calcium: 15 mg., Sodium: 8 mg., Iron: .5 mg.

B-Carotene: n/a, Vitamin C: n/a, Vitamin E: .7 mg.

Selenium: .038 mg., Zinc: .7 mg.

NUT MILK

preparation time: 10 min.

servings: 1

❑ In a nut or coffee grinder, grind the almonds as finely as possible. Place the ground almonds in a blender with the water.

❑ Run the blender at high speed for 2 minutes. Strain the resulting liquid through a very fine strainer.

Hint: If blanched almonds are used, the liquid does not need to be strained.

2 oz. almonds, finely ground (1/4 cup)
1 cup water

All information is per serving:

Calories: 150 (17% from protein, 71% from fat)
Protein: 6.9 gm., Fat: 13 gm., Linoleic Acid: n/a, Fiber: 2.5 gm.
Calcium: 102 mg., Sodium: 3.5 mg., Iron: 1.4 mg.
B-Carotene: n/a, Vitamin C: n/a, Vitamin E: n/a
Selenium: n/a, Zinc: 1.2 mg.

SPECIAL TREATS

RUTH'S YAM PEACH PIE

preparation time: 40 min.
cooking time: 60 min.

servings: 8

Polenta Crust:
1/2 cup water
1 1/2 cups apple juice
1/2 cup white or yellow cornmeal
1 tsp. cinnamon

Filling:
2 cups baked yams (approximately 1 large yam)
1 Tbsp. peach juice (or apple, orange, etc.)
1 tsp. cinnamon
2 cups diced fresh peaches (approximately 2 peaches)

❑ To make the crust, bring the water and apple juice to a boil, and slowly stir in the cornmeal and cinnamon. Continue stirring until the liquid is absorbed and the polenta becomes quite thick (about 20 minutes). Remove from the heat.

❑ Spoon the polenta into a glass pie plate. Let cool until it can be pressed into a crust. For a crisper crust, bake at 425° F for 10-15 minutes. Poke a fork into the bottom of the crust if it bubbles up.

❑ To make the filling, remove the skin from the cooked yams, and purée in a food processor with the fruit juice and cinnamon.

❑ Chop the peaches and put into a large bowl. Add the yam purée and stir well.

❑ Preheat the oven to 350° F. Pour the filling into the crust, and smooth over the top with the spoon. Bake for 20 minutes. Allow to cool completely before slicing.

Variations: In place of the peaches, try 2 cups sliced bananas or 2 cups pumpkin, puréed with the yams.

All information is per serving:

Calories: 110 (5% from protein, 3% from fat)
Protein: 1.5 gm., Fat: .4 gm., Linoleic Acid: .2 gm., Fiber: 2.8 gm.
Calcium: 18 mg., Sodium: 7.4 mg., Iron: .9 mg.
B-Carotene: 558 µg., Vitamin C: 8 mg., Vitamin E: 1.6 mg.
Selenium: .001 mg., Zinc: .3 mg.

APPLESAUCE MUFFINS

preparation time: 15 min.
cooking time: 20 min.

servings: 12

- ❑ Preheat the oven to 350° F. Mix the dry ingredients in a large bowl.

- ❑ In a separate bowl or a food processor, mix the applesauce and juice with a fork.

- ❑ Slowly add the dry ingredients, and stir together until the dry ingredients are just moistened. Fold in the raisins and diced apple.

- ❑ In a nonstick muffin tin, fill the cups to 2/3 full. Bake for 10-12 minutes. Cool and serve.

1 cup oat flour (can be oatmeal ground in a blender or food processor)
1 cup rice flour
1 tsp. baking soda
1/2 tsp. baking powder
1/2 Tbsp. cinnamon
1/4 tsp. nutmeg

1 cup applesauce
3/4 cup apple juice
1/2 cup raisins
1 apple, peeled, cored, and diced

All information is per serving:

Calories: 149 (9% from protein, 8% from fat)
Protein: 3.7 gm., Fat: 1.4 gm., Linoleic Acid: .5 gm., Fiber: 2.8 gm.
Calcium: 30 mg., Sodium: 108 mg., Iron: 1.3 mg.
B-Carotene: 1 µg., Vitamin C: 3 mg., Vitamin E: .4 mg.
Selenium: .008 mg., Zinc: .9 mg.

STRAWBERRY BANANA BREAD

preparation time: 20 min.
cooking time: 60 min.

servings: 8

2 pints fresh strawberries
3 bananas, mashed

4 cups oat flour (can be oatmeal
  ground in a blender or food
  processor)
1/2 tsp. cinnamon
1/4 tsp. allspice
2 1/2 tsp. baking powder

❑ Preheat the oven to 300° F. Juice the strawberries in a juicer to make 1 cup of juice, or blend in a blender and strain. Blend the bananas and strawberry juice in a food processor until smooth.

❑ Mix the dry ingredients in a medium mixing bowl, and add to the food processor in 2 batches, blending each time until just mixed.

❑ Pour into a nonstick loaf pan. Sprinkle a few rolled oats on top, if you like. Bake for 60 minutes. Allow to cool completely before slicing.

All information is per serving:

Calories: 214 (13% from protein, 12% from fat)
Protein: 7.3 gm., Fat: 3.0 gm., Linoleic Acid: 1.0 gm., Fiber: 5.5 gm.
Calcium: 102 mg., Sodium: 4 mg., Iron: 2.2 mg.
B-Carotene: 2 µg., Vitamin C: 36 mg., Vitamin E: .2 mg.
Selenium: .001 mg., Zinc: 1.4 mg.

TAPIOCA PUDDING

preparation time: 10 min.
cooking time: 15 min.
cooling time: 20 min.

servings: 4

❑ In a blender, blend the banana, dates, and rice milk or juice. Pour into a 2-quart saucepan, and add the tapioca. Let it stand for 5 minutes.

❑ Cook on medium heat until it reaches a full boil, stirring constantly. Remove from the heat. Stir in the vanilla.

❑ Allow to cool about 20 minutes. (It will thicken as it cools.) Serve warm or chilled.

1 banana
2 Tbsp. pitted, chopped dates, (8 dates)
2 1/2 cups Rice Milk (see p. 151) or fruit juice
3 Tbsp. quick-cooking tapioca

1 tsp. vanilla extract (alcohol-free)

All information is per serving:

Calories: 130 (5% from protein, 4% from fat)
Protein: 1.8 gm., Fat: .7 gm., Linoleic Acid: .2 gm., Fiber: 1.9 gm.
Calcium: 11 mg., Sodium: 1 mg., Iron: .6 mg.
B-Carotene: n/a, Vitamin C: 3 mg., Vitamin E: .5 mg.
Selenium: .024 mg., Zinc: .5 mg.

SWEET YAM PUDDING

preparation time: 20 min.

servings: 8

4 large oranges
4 large yams, baked and peeled
1 tsp. cinnamon
1/4 tsp. nutmeg

❑ Juice the oranges, saving both the juice and the orange halves.

❑ In the food processor, blend the yams, spices, and just enough orange juice to whip them to a fluffy consistency.

❑ Lightly spoon back into the orange shells. Top with a sprinkle of cinnamon or a sprig of fresh mint. Serve warm or chilled.

All information is per serving:
Calories: 90 (7% from protein, 2% from fat)
Protein: 1.6 gm., Fat: .2 gm., Linoleic Acid: .04 gm., Fiber: 3.3 gm.
Calcium: 46 mg., Sodium: 5.8 mg., Iron: .4 mg.
B-Carotene: 1243 µg., Vitamin C: 49 mg., Vitamin E: 2.8 mg.
Selenium: .002 mg., Zinc: .2 mg.

FRUIT POLENTA SQUAR

preparation time: 20 min.
cooking time: 25 min.
cooling time: 30 min.

servings: 18 squares

❑ Bring the water and juice to a boil in a 2-quart saucepan. Add the cornmeal and reduce the heat to medium, stirring to mix well.

❑ Add the remaining ingredients and cook for 5 more minutes, stirring constantly, until thick.

❑ Preheat the oven to 300° F. Spread into an 8-inch x 8-inch nonstick baking dish, and bake for 20-25 minutes. Cool and cut into squares.

1 cup water
3 cups juice (pear, apple, grape, etc.)
1 cup white or yellow cornmeal

6 dates, pitted and chopped
1/2 cup raisins
1/2 tsp. cinnamon

All information is per serving:

Calories: 64 (5% from protein, 4% from fat)

Protein: .8 gm., Fat: .3 gm., Linoleic Acid: .1 gm., Fiber: 1.5 gm.

Calcium: 7 mg., Sodium: 4.5 mg., Iron: .5 mg.

B-Carotene: n/a, Vitamin C: .5 mg., Vitamin E: .1 mg.

Selenium: .001 mg., Zinc: .2 mg.

OATMEAL RAISIN COOKIES

preparation time: 20 min.
cooking time: 10 min.

servings: 12

4 cups oat flour (can be oatmeal
ground in a blender or food
processor)
1 tsp. baking powder
1/2 tsp. baking soda
1 tsp. cinnamon
1/4 tsp. nutmeg

2 ripe bananas, mashed
1 cup apple juice

1/2 cup raisins

❑ Preheat the oven to 375° F. Mix the dry
ingredients in a large bowl.

❑ In a food processor, blend the bananas
and juice until smooth.

❑ Slowly add the dry ingredients while
mixing.

❑ Pour the batter into the large bowl, and
add the raisins. Drop by spoonfuls onto
a nonstick baking sheet. Bake for 10
minutes.

All information is per serving:

Calories: 249 (14% from protein, 13% from fat)
Protein: 9.2 gm., Fat: 3.8 gm., Linoleic Acid: 1.3 gm., Fiber: 7.6 gm.
Calcium: 54 mg., Sodium: 55 mg., Iron: 2.8 mg.
B-Carotene: n/a, Vitamin C: 2 mg., Vitamin E: .7 mg.
Selenium: .015 mg., Zinc: 2.1 mg.

WHEAT-FREE BARS

preparation time: 15 min.
cooking time: 10 min.

servings: 12

☐ Preheat the oven to 350° F. In a food processor, combine the bananas, juice, and water until smooth.

☐ Add the oat flour slowly while mixing, and press into an 8-inch x 8-inch non-stick baking dish.

☐ Bake for 10 minutes. Cool and cut into bars with a hard plastic spatula.

4 ripe bananas, mashed
1 1/2 cups peach or plum juice, or 1 cup apple juice concentrate
1/2 cup water

3 cups oat flour (can be oatmeal ground in a blender or food processor)

All information is per serving:

Calories: 265 (11% from protein, 10% from fat)
Protein: 7.4 gm., Fat: 3.0 gm., Linoleic Acid: 1.0 gm., Fiber: 6.7 gm.
Calcium: 36 mg., Sodium: 8.2 mg., Iron: 2.5 mg.
B-Carotene: n/a, Vitamin C: 35 mg., Vitamin E: .6 mg.
Selenium: .011 mg., Zinc: 1.7 mg.

DATE COCONUT PIE

preparation time: 20 min.
chilling time: 2 hours

servings: 8

1 1/2 cups grated fresh coconut
1 cup any fruit juice

3 large bananas
2/3 cup whole pitted dates

2/3 cup shredded coconut
1/3 cup pitted, sliced dates

❑ Moisten the grated fresh coconut with the juice, and pat into a glass pie plate for a crust. Chill.

❑ Meanwhile, mix the bananas and whole pitted dates in a blender with just enough water so they will combine easily (the mixture should be quite thick). Pour over the crust.

❑ Top with the shredded coconut and sliced, pitted dates. Chill for at least 2 hours.

All information is per serving:

Calories: 240 (3% from protein, 32% from fat)
Protein: 1.6 gm., Fat: 9.3 gm., Linoleic Acid: .2 gm., Fiber: 3.8 gm.
Calcium: 15 mg., Sodium: 68 mg., Iron: 1.0 mg.
B-Carotene: n/a, Vitamin C: 4 mg., Vitamin E: .3 mg.
Selenium: .005 mg., Zinc: .6 mg.

APPLE PIE

preparation time: 30 min.
cooking time: 25 min.

servings: 8

❑ To make the crust, mix the oat flour and juice, and knead into a dough. Pat out into a pie plate.

❑ Bring all the filling ingredients to a boil in a large saucepan. Simmer for 20 minutes.

❑ Preheat the oven to 350° F. Pour the apple filling into the pie crust, sprinkle with additional cinnamon, and bake for 10 minutes. Let cool before serving.

Variation: Replace 4 apples with 10 ounces of frozen blueberries. Add the blueberries after cooking for 15 minutes; finish cooking for 10 more minutes.

Crust:
2 1/2 cups oat flour (can be oatmeal ground in a blender or food processor)
1 cup apple juice

Filling:
6 baking apples, peeled, cored, and sliced
3/4 cup apple juice
1 Tbsp. lemon juice
1/2 tsp. cinnamon
1/4 tsp. nutmeg

All information is per serving:

Calories: 278 (12% from protein, 12% from fat)
Protein: 8.4 gm., Fat: 3.8 gm., Linoleic Acid: 2.3 gm., Fiber: 8 gm.
Calcium: 37 mg., Sodium: 3 mg., Iron: 2.7 mg.
B-Carotene: 5 μg., Vitamin C: 5 mg., Vitamin E: .8 mg.
Selenium: .015 mg., Zinc: 2 mg.

FROZEN BLUEBERRY PIE

preparation time: 20 min.
chilling time: 2 hours

servings: 8

Crust:
2 cups walnuts
1 1/2 cups unsweetened shredded coconut
3/4 cup apple juice

Filling:
4 cups fresh or frozen blueberries (10 oz.)
5 dates, finely sliced
1/2 cup apple juice

❑ To make the crust, place all the crust ingredients in a food processor or blender, and purée until well mixed. Spread into a glass pie dish, covering the bottom and sides evenly. Cover and chill in the refrigerator while preparing the filling.

❑ To make the filling, place all the filling ingredients in a food processor or blender, and purée until smooth. Pour into the crust, smoothing it evenly with a spatula. Cover the pie and return it to the freezer until firm (about 2 hours).

All information is per serving:

Calories: 352 (6% from protein, 61% from fat)
Protein: 5.3 gm., Fat: 25.3 gm., Linoleic Acid: 9.6 gm., Fiber: 4.9 gm.
Calcium: 41 mg., Sodium: 50.1 mg., Iron: 1.4 mg.
B-Carotene: 9.8 µg., Vitamin C: 3 mg., Vitamin E: 1.7 mg.
Selenium: .009 mg., Zinc: 1.2 mg.

VEGETABLE-OAT BREAD

preparation time: 30 min.
cooking time: 45 min.

servings: 8

❑ In a large bowl, mix the yams and water or juice with a fork until well blended.

❑ In a separate bowl, mix the oats, baking soda, baking powder, cinnamon, and nutmeg.

❑ Slowly stir the dry mixture into the yam mixture. Add the carrots and zucchini, and mix well.

❑ Preheat the oven to 350° F. Spoon into a glass loaf pan, and bake for 45 minutes. Cover with aluminum foil for the first 25 minutes. Allow to cool before slicing.

Variation: Add 3 Tbsp. grated fresh ginger.

1/2 cup cooked, peeled yams
1 cup water or apple/celery juice made from 3 ribs celery, 1 apple, or juice of 1 lemon

4 cups oat flour (can be oatmeal ground in a blender or food processor)
2 tsp. baking soda
1 tsp. baking powder
1 tsp. cinnamon
1/4 tsp. nutmeg

1/2 cup shredded carrots
1/2 cup shredded zucchini

All information is per serving:

Calories: 376 (15% from protein, 14% from fat)

Protein: 14.2 gm., Fat: 6.0 gm., Linoleic Acid: 1.9 gm., Fiber: 14.6 gm.

Calcium: 96 mg., Sodium: 350 mg., Iron: 4.8 mg.

B-Carotene: 224 µg., Vitamin C: 21 mg., Vitamin E: 2.0 mg.

Selenium: .022 mg., Zinc: 3.3 mg.

ROZEN BANANA DELIGHT

preparation time: 15 min.

servings: 3

6 ripe bananas

❑ Peel the ripe bananas and place in a single layer in a sealed plastic bag; freeze overnight.

❑ At least 15 minutes before preparing, place any removable parts from your juicer (including the blank or solid juicer plate) in the freezer, along with a serving bowl. Chilling these parts will keep the bananas from melting too quickly when processed. Reassemble the juicer and place the bowl at the open end of the machine.

❑ Break the bananas in half, and push through the juicer with the plunger. Serve immediately; this does not refreeze well. May be topped with fresh berries or fat-free granola.

Hint: This can be made in a blender, but the texture will not be as smooth and creamy.

All information is per serving:

Calories: 210 (4% from protein, 4% from fat)

Protein: 2.4 gm., Fat: 1.1 gm., Linoleic Acid: .1 gm., Fiber: 3.9 gm.

Calcium: 14 mg., Sodium: 2 mg., Iron: .7 mg.

B-Carotene: n/a, Vitamin C: 21 mg., Vitamin E: .6 mg.

Selenium: .002 mg., Zinc: .4 mg.

QUICK PEACH BETTY

preparation time: 20 min.
cooking time: 30 min.

servings: 4

6 ripe peaches, sliced
3 cups fresh raspberries or sliced strawberries
1 cup oil-free granola
1 cup apple juice

❑ Preheat the oven to 350° F. Layer the peaches and berries in a 2-quart baking dish, and top with the granola. Sprinkle the juice over the top to moisten the granola.

❑ Bake uncovered for about 30 minutes, or until the peaches are tender. Can be served warm or chilled.

Variations: Great topped with Frozen Banana Delight (see p. 166). Try plums instead of peaches.

All information is per serving:

Calories: 282 (11% from protein, 10% from fat)
Protein: 8.4 gm., Fat: 3.4 gm., Linoleic Acid: 1.2 gm., Fiber: 11.5 gm.
Calcium: 52 mg., Sodium: 2.5 mg., Iron: 2.7 mg.
B-Carotene: n/a, Vitamin C: 32 mg., Vitamin E: .8 mg.
Selenium: .013 mg., Zinc: 2.2 mg.

APPLE JACK BREAD

preparation time: 30 min.
cooking time: 45 min.

servings: 8

5 apples, peeled, cored, and quartered
1 cup raisins
1 cup water or apple-celery juice
1 Tbsp. lemon juice
1 tsp. cinnamon
1/2 tsp. nutmeg
1/4 tsp. cloves

2 cups oat flour (can be oatmeal ground in a blender or food processor)
1 tsp. baking soda
1 Tbsp. baking powder

❑ In a 2-quart saucepan, combine the apples, raisins, water, lemon juice, and spices.

❑ Cook over medium heat until the apples are tender and the liquid is reduced by half. Set aside until cooled.

❑ Preheat the oven to 350° F.

❑ Combine the remaining dry ingredients in a separate mixing bowl.

❑ Combine the dry mixture with the cooled apple mixture. Pour the batter into an 8-inch, nonstick loaf pan. Cover for the first 30 minutes of cooking with aluminum foil.

❑ Bake for about 45 minutes, or until a toothpick inserted in the middle of the loaf comes out clean.

All information is per serving:

Calories: 256 (11% from protein, 10% from fat)
Protein: 7.3 gm., Fat: 3.1 gm., Linoleic Acid: 1.0 gm., Fiber: 7.2 gm.
Calcium: 119 mg., Sodium: 163 mg., Iron: 2.6 mg.
B-Carotene: 4 µg., Vitamin C: 4.8 mg., Vitamin E: .8 mg.
Selenium: .011 mg., Zinc: 1.7 mg.

BANANA BREAD

preparation time: 20 min.
cooking time: 45 min.

servings: 8

- ❑ Blend the bananas and juice in a blender or food processor until smooth.

- ❑ In a separate bowl, mix the dry ingredients well.

- ❑ Preheat the oven to 350° F.

- ❑ Add the dry mixture to the bananas while processing, or pour the blended bananas in a separate bowl, and mix the dry ingredients in by hand.

- ❑ Pour into a glass loaf pan, and bake for 45 minutes, covering with aluminum foil for the first 25 minutes.

Variation: Replace the apple juice with the juice of 1 apple, 4 large strawberries, and 3 ribs of celery. You can also add raisins or sliced dates to the final batter.

4 ripe bananas
1 cup apple juice
juice of 1 lemon

4 cups oat flour (can be oatmeal ground in a blender or food processor)
2 tsp. baking soda
1 tsp. baking powder
2 tsp. cinnamon
1/4 tsp. nutmeg or allspice

All information is per serving:

Calories: 375 (14% from protein, 13% from fat)
Protein: 13.9 gm., Fat: 5.8 gm., Linoleic Acid: 1.9 gm., Fiber: 11.5 gm.
Calcium: 84 mg., Sodium: 318 mg., Iron: 4.3 mg.
B-Carotene: n/a, Vitamin C: 9.4 mg., Vitamin E: n/a
Selenium: .022 mg., Zinc: 3.2 mg.

STUFFED BAKED APPLES

preparation time: 30 min.
cooking time: 45 min.

servings: 6

1 cup pitted, chopped dates
2 cups apple juice

1 cup rolled oat flour (can be oatmeal ground in a blender or food processor)
2 tsp. cinnamon
1 tsp. nutmeg
1/2 tsp. ginger

6 apples, cored, leaving the base intact

❑ In a 1-quart saucepan, combine the dates and 1 cup of the apple juice, and simmer for 30 minutes, or until the liquid is reduced by half.

❑ Mix the oats, cinnamon, nutmeg, and ginger in a mixing bowl. Add to the date mixture, and mix well.

❑ Preheat the oven to 350° F.

❑ Place the apples upright in a baking dish, and fill with the date/oat mixture. Pour the remaining 1 cup of apple juice over the apples.

❑ Bake uncovered for 45 minutes, or until the apples are tender.

All information is per serving:

Calories: 299 (7% from protein, 7% from fat)
Protein: 5.3 gm., Fat: 2.6 gm., Linoleic Acid: .8 gm., Fiber: 8.1 gm.
Calcium: 44 mg., Sodium: 4 mg., Iron: 2.3 mg.
B-Carotene: 6.4 µg., Vitamin C: 6.1 mg., Vitamin E: .6 mg.
Selenium: .009 mg., Zinc: 1.2 mg.

APPLESAUCE

preparation time: 20 min.
cooking time: 30 min.

servings: 24 ounces

❑ In a heavy-bottomed 4-quart saucepan, combine the apples, raisins, water, and mint leaves.

❑ Cover and cook over low heat for 30 minutes, adding more water as needed to maintain desired thickness and to avoid sticking.

❑ Remove from the heat and blend in a food processor until smooth. If you desire an even smoother texture, press through a fine strainer.

Variation: Add 1 tsp. cinnamon and/or 1/2 tsp. nutmeg once blended.

12 apples, peeled, cored, and diced
1/2 cup raisins
1/2 cup water
8 fresh mint leaves (optional)

All information is per serving:

Calories: 273 (2% from protein, 4% from fat)

Protein: 1.2 gm., Fat: 1.3 gm., Linoleic Acid: .3 gm., Fiber: 6.5 gm.

Calcium: 25 mg., Sodium: 3 mg., Iron: .6 mg.

B-Carotene: 19 µg., Vitamin C: 16 mg., Vitamin E: 1.2 mg.

Selenium: .003 mg., Zinc: .2 mg.

A WELL-EQUIPPED KITCHEN

STORAGE

12 1 qt. or 2 qt. Glass Jars
25 4oz Glass Bottles for herbs
"Ziplock" Freezer Bags
Glass or Plastic Storage Containers
    four   3 qt.
    one   2 qt.
    one   1 qt. bottle

POTS 'N PANS

Steamer Pot (10 qt.)
Soup/Stock Pot (10 qt.)
Saucepan with Lid (6 qt.)
1-2 Saucepans with Lid (2 qt.)
Sauté Pan with Lid (1 qt.)
Nonstick Griddle/Fry Pan
Casserole Dish with Lid
9" x 13" Glass Baking Dish
Nonstick Baking Pans:
Muffin Tin
2 Cookie Sheets
2 Cake Pans
2 Loaf Pans

HANDY APPLIANCES

Food Processor
Blender
Juicer
Nut Grinder
Hand Mixer
Toaster Oven

TOOLS AND UTENSILS

Wooden Cutting Board
8"-10" Chef's Knife
Straightening Steel
3" Paring Knife
Vegetable Peeler
Wire Whisk
2 Wooden Spoons
Serving Spoon
Ladle
Tongs
Spatula
Potato Masher
1 Very Large Metal Mixing Bowl
2 Medium Metal Mixing Bowls
2 Cup Glass Measuring Cup
  (for liquids)
1 Cup Glass Measuring Cup
Set of Nested Plastic Measuring
  Cups
Measuring Spoons
Colander
Lettuce Spinner

FOR EATING

Large Bowls for Salad

FOODS USED IN THE HEALTH PROMOTING COOKBOOK

FRUIT

Apples:
    Fuji
    Gata
    Golden Delicious
    Granny Smith
    Red Delicious
Apricots
Bananas
Blueberries
Figs
Grapes
Grapefruits
Kiwis
Lemons
Mangoes
Melons:
    Cantaloupe
    Honeydew
    Watermelon
Nectarines
Oranges
Peaches
Pears:
    Asian
    Bosc
    Comice
Pineapples
Plums
Raspberries
Strawberries
Tangerines

VEGETABLES

Alfalfa Sprouts
Arugula
Artichokes
Asparagus
Avocado
Bean Sprouts
Beets
Belgian Endive
Bell Peppers
Bok Choy
Brussel Sprouts
Broccoli
Cabbage:
    Chinese
    Red
    Green
Carrots
Celery
Chard:
    Green
    Red
Ancho Chilis (mild)
Corn
Cucumbers
Eggplant
Green Beans
Jicama
Kale
Leeks
Lettuce:
    Red Leaf
    Romaine

VEGETABLES (CONTINUED)

Mushrooms
Okra
Onions:
   Green
   Red
   Yellow
Parsnips
Peas:
   English
   Snap
   Snow
Potatoes:
   Purple
   Red
   Russet
   Yukon Gold
Rutabagas
Shallots
Spinach
Squash:
   Acorn
   Butternut
   Spaghetti
   Crookneck
   Zucchini
Sweet Potatoes
Tomatoes
Turnips
Yams

FLOURS

Cornmeal
Oat

WHOLE GRAINS

Amaranth
Brown Rice
   Black Japonica
   Basmati
   Short Grain
   Sweet
Wild Millet
Oats
Cornmeal
Quinoa

LEGUMES (BEANS)

Black
Black-eyed Peas
Garbanzo
Lima
Lentils
   Brown
   Red
Navy
Pinto
White
Split Peas
   Green
   Yellow

DRIED FRUIT

(unsulphered) Currants
Dates
Figs
Papaya
Raisins
Shredded Coconut
Sundried Tomatoes

HERBS AND SPICES

Allspice
Arrowroot
Bay Leaves
Cardamom
Celery Seed
Chervil Chives
Cilantro
Cinnamon Powder
Ginger
Italian Seasonings
Marjoram
Mint
Mustard
Nutmeg Powder
Orange Zest
Oregano
Parsley
Rosemary
Sage
Savory
Star Anise
Tarragon
Thyme
Turmeric

NUTS AND SEEDS

Almonds
Cashews
Pecans
Pumpkin Seeds
Sesame Seeds
Sunflower Seeds
Walnuts

PACKAGED ITEMS

Apple Cider Vinegar
Baking Soda (non-aluminum)
Baking Powder
Oil-Free Salad Dressing
Corn Pasta
Corn Tortillas
Dulse
Tapioca (instant)
Tofu
Tomato Paste (salt-free)
Vanilla (alcohol-free)

PREPARATION OF BEANS

PROPORTIONS BEAN	COOKING LIQUID/BEAN	TIME
BROWN LENTILS	1 1/2:1	30-45 min.
RED LENTILS	2:1	20-30 min.

Procedure: Rinse well. Bring the liquid and lentils to a boil, reduce the heat to a simmer, cover, and cook.

SPLIT PEAS	1 1/2:1	1 hour 30 min. (green and yellow)

Procedure: Rinse well. Bring the liquid and lentils to a boil, reduce the heat to a simmer, cover, and cook.

BLACK BEANS	2:1	2 hours
BLACK-EYED PEAS	2:1	60 min.
GARBANZO BEANS	3:1	4 hours 30 min.
LIMA BEANS	2:1	60 min.
PINTO BEANS	2:1	2 hours
WHITE BEANS	2:1	2 hours

Procedure: Rinse well. Bring the liquid to a vigorous boil for 3 to 4 min., then drain the water. This will eliminate much of the indigestible starch that helps contribute to excess gas. Cover the beans with fresh liquid, and bring to a boil. Reduce the heat to a simmer, cover, and cook.

PREPARATION OF GRAINS

GRAIN	PROPORTIONS LIQUID/GRAIN	COOKING TIME
BROWN RICE	1 1/2:1	45 min.

Procedure: Bring the liquid to a boil. Add the brown rice, return to a boil, then cover, and simmer for 45 min. Remove from the heat; let stand covered for 15 min. Remove the lid and fluff with a fork.

MILLET	2:1	30 min.

Procedure: Bring the liquid to a boil. Add the millet, return to a boil, then cover, and simmer for 30 min.

CORNMEAL (for stovetop)	4:1	20 min.

Procedure: Bring the liquid to a boil. Add the cornmeal and return to a low boil. Stir constantly with a wire whisk until the polenta starts to pull away from the pan. Eat warm or allow to cool in a mold.

CORNMEAL (for oven)	3:1	5 min. plus 60 min.

Procedure: Bring the liquid to a boil. Add the cornmeal and return to a low boil. Stir constantly with a wire whisk for 5 min. Transfer the polenta to a baking dish, cover, and bake at 350°F for 60 min. or until done.

QUINOA	1 1/2:1	20 min.

Procedure: Rinse well and drain as much water as possible. Bring the liquid to a boil, add the quinoa, and return to a boil. Cover and simmer for 20 min. Fluff with a fork.

OATS (quick)	2:1	5 min.
OATS (rolled)	2:1	20 min.

Procedure: Bring the liquid and oats to a boil. Reduce to a simmer and stir constantly. Adjust the liquid and cooking time for desired consistency.

BARLEY	3:1	40 min.

Procedure: Rinse the barley. Bring the water to a boil, add the barley, and return to a boil. Lower the heat to a simmer, cover, and cook.

About the Center

The TrueNorth Health Center, operates a residential health care program in northern California. Founded in 1984, this 17 bed facility is located on two acres in a country setting in Penngrove, California, just 10 minutes south of Santa Rosa and one hour north of San Francisco.

The Center has a staff of seven doctors specializing in the supervision of therapeutic fasting and in helping people to make diet and lifestyle changes. The Center also operates an out-patient clinic called the TrueNorth Health Clinic.

If you would like to receive our complimentary newsletter or an information packet about the Center programs, write:

TrueNorth Health Center
6010 Commerce Blvd. #152
Rohnert Park, CA 94928
or call the Center
(707) 586-5555
www.healthpromoting.com

If you need help with a specific health concern, consult with a doctor trained in health promotion. For a doctor in your area, call:

TrueNorth Health Clinic
(707) 586-5555

About the Author

Dr. Alan Goldhamer, the founder and director of the TrueNorth Health Center, is the author of *The Health Promoting Cookbook*. Dr. Goldhamer is an expert in the use of diet and lifestyle modification in helping individuals learn to achieve and maintain optimum health. The recipes in this book were developed by the staff of the residential health care program at the TrueNorth Health Center. Special thanks go to Mary Carpenter, Kathy Ballard, Ruth Tipler, Sienna Hornback, Elaine Garcia, and Cybele Bantowky.

Highly Recommended

The American Natural Hygiene Society is a national, nonprofit health education organization providing on-going information and support through their award-winning magazine *Health Science*. To become a member or get more information, contact:

American Natural Hygiene Society
P.O. Box 30630
Tampa, FL 33630
phone (813) 855-6607
fax (813) 855-8052
email: anhs@anhs.org
Internet: http://anhs.org

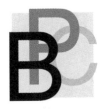

BOOK PUBLISHING COMPANY

since 1974—books that educate, inspire, and empower

Visit BookPubCo.com to find your favorite books on plant-based cooking and nutrition, raw foods, and healthy living.

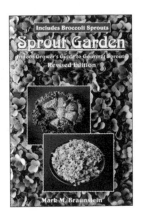

Sprout Garden

Indoor Grower's Guide to Gourmet Sprouts
Mark M. Braunstein

This easy-to-use guide provides information on how to grow sprouts at home, the best growing technique for each tupe of sprout, health information on alfalfa sprouts and broccoli sprouts, sources for sprouting equipment and seeds, and a great collection of delicious recipes.

978-1-57067-073-2
$12.95

Purchase this health title from your local bookstore or natural food store, or you can buy it directly from:

Book Publishing Company
P.O. Box 99
Summertown, TN 38483
1-888-260-8458

Free shipping and handling on all book orders.

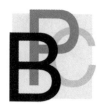
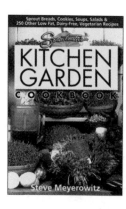

Sproutman's Kitchen Garden Cookbook

Steve Meyerowitz

Turn nuts, vegetable seeds, grains, and beans into gourmet food. Includes recipes for sprout breads, cookies, crackers, soups, pizza, bagels, dressings, dips, spreads, sautés, nondairy milks, and ice creams. Also, food dehydrating, juicing, natural sodas, and foods glossary.

978-1-87873-686-4
$14.95

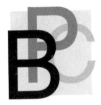

BOOK PUBLISHING COMPANY

since 1974—books that educate, inspire, and empower

Visit BookPubCo.com to find your favorite books on plant-based cooking and nutrition, raw foods, and healthy living.

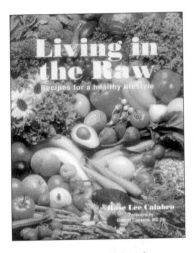

Purchase this health title from your local bookstore or natural food store, or you can buy it directly from:

Book Publishing Company
P.O. Box 99
Summertown, TN 38483
1-888-260-8458

Free shipping and handling on all book orders.

Living in the Raw

Recipes for a Healthy Lifestyle
Rose Lee Calabro

Follow easy suggestions for how to sprout and dehydrate a host of beans, grains, and seeds and use them in conjunction with fruits, vegetables, herbs, and spices to create nutritious, healing foods.

Over 300 recipes are given for everything from breads, crackers, cakes, and ice cream to appetizers, hearty main dishes, and soups. Includes sections on setting up a living foods kitchen and why a raw foods diet will help anyone feel great and look great.

978-1-57067-148-7
$19.95

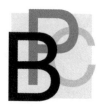

BOOK PUBLISHING COMPANY

since 1974—books that educate, inspire, and empower
Visit BookPubCo.com to find your favorite books on plant-based cooking and nutrition, raw foods, and healthy living.

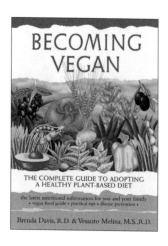

Purchase this health title from your local bookstore or natural food store, or you can buy it directly from:

Book Publishing Company
P.O. Box 99
Summertown, TN 38483
1-888-260-8458

Free shipping and handling on all book orders.

Becoming Vegan

The Complete Guide to Adopting a Healthy Plant-Based Diet
Brenda Davis, R.D. & Vesanto Melina, M.S., R.D

Two of North America's foremost vegetarian dietitians present up-to-date findings on:

- How a vegan diet can protect against cancer, and heart disease
- Getting enough protein without meat
- Meeting calcium needs without dairy products
- Balanced vegan diets for infants, children, and seniors
- Pregnancy and breast-feeding tips for vegan moms

978-1-57067-103-6
$19.95

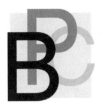
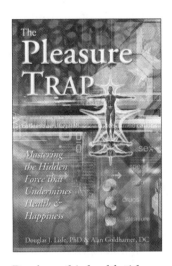

Cuecurmin
= Flat

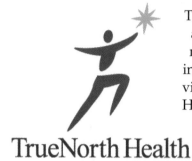

TrueNorth Health

The TrueNorth Health Center has operated a residential health education program in northern California since 1984. This live-in program specializes in medically supervised fasting. The doctors at TrueNorth Health have had the results of their research published in peer-reviewed scientific journals.

You can learn more about the Center, read the results of our research, check out health-promoting recipes, and sign up for our free newsletter by visiting our web site. You may also write to us and have your questions answered by Dr. Goldhamer online.

Visit out web site at www.healthpromoting.com or telephone the TrueNorth Health Center at (707) 586-5555.